Patients and Social Practice of Psychiatric Nursing in the 19th and 20th Century

T0139531

Medizin,
Gesellschaft und Geschichte

Jahrbuch
des Instituts für Geschichte der Medizin
der Robert Bosch Stiftung

herausgegeben von
Robert Jütte

Beiheft 66

Patients and Social Practice of Psychiatric Nursing in the 19th and 20th Century

Edited by Sylvelyn Hähner-Rombach and Karen Nolte

Franz Steiner Verlag Stuttgart
2017

Gedruckt mit freundlicher Unterstützung der Robert Bosch Stiftung GmbH

Coverabbildung:
Badesaal für unruhige Frauen
aus: „Deutsche Heil- und Pflegeanstalten für Psychischkranke in Wort und Bild",
S. 158; Carl Marhold Verlagsbuchhandlung, Halle a. S., 1910

Bibliografische Information der Deutschen Nationalbibliothek:
Die Deutsche Nationalbibliothek verzeichnet diese Publikation in der Deutschen
Nationalbibliografie; detaillierte bibliografische Daten sind im Internet über
<http://dnb.d-nb.de> abrufbar.

© Franz Steiner Verlag, Stuttgart 2017
Druck: Laupp & Göbel GmbH, Gomaringen
Gedruckt auf säurefreiem, alterungsbeständigem Papier.
Printed in Germany
ISBN 978-3-515-11716-6 (Print)
ISBN 978-3-515-11718-0 (E-Book)

Contents

Reform and Training of Psychiatric Nurses

Introduction: Patients and Social Practice of Psychiatric Nursing in the 19th and 20th Century

Karen Nolte / Sylvelyn Hähner-Rombach

In the last twenty years, the history of psychiatry has developed into an area of research characterised by multidisciplinary perspectives and questions. At first, historians tackled questions of psychiatry as a profession, as a science and as an institution. In the 1980s and 90s, the psychiatric hospital was principally regarded as a social disciplinary institution, thus emphasising the link between the interests of medicine and state order. The early phase of socio-historical research into psychiatry was dominated by the perspective of authority and the psychiatrist towards psychiatry and thus also the patients.[1] This was overlapped by scientific history questions, such as the social construction of illness, which seemed particularly appropriate in the field of psychiatry. Further scientific access was created by questions of knowledge production through psychiatric and medical case histories[2] as well as through techniques and methods of "psychiatric record taking"[3]. It is only in the last twenty years that everyday life in the hospitals and psychiatric therapies has increasingly come into the spotlight of psychiatric historians. Linked to this was the question of subjective perceptions of patients. Thus, researchers into psychiatric history followed the demand of the British medical historian Roy Porter to take a "patient's view"[4] of the history of medicine.[5]

In this research of everyday history, the history of psychiatric caregivers remained almost untouched.[6] This is particularly surprising as caregivers played a key role in psychiatric hospitals until well into the 20th century: Thus, around 1900, a doctor, depending on the hospital, was responsible for one to two hundred patients[7], i. e. patients rarely saw a doctor and doctors had to base much of their judgement on observations and the appropriate descriptions from caregivers.

The long silence in historical research on the history of psychiatric nursing is primarily due to the difficult situation with sources: Even into the 20th century, the activity of caregivers was an unskilled profession, practised by people of the lower social classes. Although the "service" provided by these

---

1 Cf. particularly the works of Dirk Blasius and Klaus Dörner, Blasius (1980) and (1994) as well as Dörner (1984), cf. also Goldberg (1999).
2 Cf. Brändli/Lüthi/Spuhler (2009).
3 Borck/Schäfer (2015).
4 Porter (1985).
5 Cf. Nolte (2013), Fuchs/Rotzoll et al. (2007), Ankele (2009), Gründler (2013).
6 An exception to this is the work of Peter Nolan, which describes the development of psychiatric nursing from the end of 19th to the end of the 20th century in England. Here, the training and working conditions and particularly reforms in psychiatry and their impacts on nursing are investigated in detail. Cf. Nolan (1993).
7 Urbach (2016).

people was an important basis for the success of psychiatric hospital therapies, the actions of caregivers were barely documented in the patient files. In addition, the approach to the everyday lives of psychiatric caregivers and their subjective perceptions in the 19th and early 20th century presents a difficult challenge, as there are very few sources handed down by the caregivers themselves.

The first German-language work in the history of psychiatric caregivers – such as the studies by Höll/Schmidt-Michel[8] and Dorothee Falkenstein[9] – initially concentrated on the virulent question of the mid-19th century, namely regarding the characteristics of a good caregiver, based on clinic and hospital rules and printed sources, which were primarily documented from the perspective of psychiatrists. Thus, normative expectations of psychiatric caregivers were reconstructed as everyday care. In her study of the history of psychiatric care in the Netherlands, Geertje Boschma showed that the establishment of psychiatry as a scientific subdiscipline of medicine was coupled with a professionalisation of psychiatric care.[10] Also, in her recently published study on the Am Steinhof sanatoria and mental hospitals in Vienna, the historian Sophie Ledebur emphasised the significance of well-trained nursing personnel for the implementation of reformist concepts in hospital psychiatry and reconstructed the processes of the professionalisation of psychiatric care in Austria using the example of this Viennese hospital.[11] Anja Faber, in her study of everyday in-patient nursing life between 1880 and 1930, published in 2015, also investigated various nursing groups in detail, including the minders of the Illenau sanatorium and mental hospital in Baden.[12] Amongst the things she investigated were the social profile of the minders, the living and working conditions, training and activities, as well as the areas of tension and conflict, including complaints about the minders.

Before this, Sabine Braunschweig, in her study of the history of psychiatric nursing in Switzerland, used the example of the Friedmatt Hospital in Basel to show how the reports written by doctors in the psychiatric patient files could be read "against the grain", thus offering a chance to find out the perspectives of nurses and nursing practices.[13] She pointed out that the reports on the social behaviour and psychiatric states of the patients in everyday ward life were primarily based on the observations of caregivers, which were forwarded to the doctors on a daily basis in reports.[14] These caregiver reports, passed on by the doctors, can thus be analysed in a careful and methodical way as a source for nursing history and, as a result, can be used to reconstruct nursing practices in psychiatry. In this way, Braunschweig has opened up the

8   Höll/Schmidt-Höll (1989).
9   Falkenstein (2000).
10   Cf. Boschma (2003).
11   Ledebur (2015), p. 97–104.
12   Faber (2015).
13   Braunschweig (2013).
14   Braunschweig (2013), p. 179–187.

path to historical research into everyday life in psychiatric nursing, particularly for the period for which no more contemporary witnesses are available. However, her appeal for further investigation of patient files of the 19th and early 20th century for patient history analyses seen from a nursing history point of view has only been pursued by very few researchers. Through her research into the Uchtspringe sanatorium and mental hospital, Anna Urbach has been able to prove an early form of specialisation in psychiatric nursing: There, caregivers were already trained in the last years of the 19th century in observing and documenting the fits of the patients diagnosed as being epileptic as accurately as possible.[15] She has also determined a decisive role of caregivers in the implementation of the concept of work therapy.[16] Sabine Braunschweig also emphasised the important role of caregivers in the introduction and evaluation of new methods of therapy in psychiatric clinics and hospitals, as the observations of the everyday life of the patients by the nursing staff were decisive in the evaluation of the effectiveness of the therapy form. In particular, during the establishment of somatic therapies, especially in electroshock therapies, the nursing personnel was essential due to their close observation of the behaviour of the patients and the controlling of vital signs – this was also shown by Gerda Engelbracht's study of the history of the nerve clinic in Bremen-Ost.[17] She has dedicated a whole chapter to the history of the nursing personnel and supplemented the archive sources from the clinic's history with interviews with former caregivers. In her second study, on the history of the Alsterdorfer Anstalten in Hamburg, which was also carried out with Andrea Hauser, the author also dedicates an extensive chapter to nursing and describes – again with reference to contemporary witness interviews – the special situation of caregivers in the setup of the deaconry between the Christian understanding of caregiving and the demands for the professionalisation of the nursing profession in the post-war years in Germany.[18]

That so-called oral history in the reconstruction of the history of psychiatric nursing is so decisive can also be seen in current research. An early example are interviews carried out with the employees of the Psychiatric Nerve Clinic of the Charité hospital in Berlin.[19] Currently, due to the difficult situation with sources, it is primarily the second half of the 20th century which is the focus of nursing history research, as there is not only a more comprehensive set of sources from the psychiatric caregivers themselves, but also the possibility of holding narrative, autobiographical interviews with contemporary witnesses, thus allowing the reconstruction of subjective perceptions and the everyday practices of psychiatric caregivers. The method of oral history was considered a major problem by historians during its rise in the early 1980s, as recollections become more unreliable over time, as the subjects,

---

15   Urbach (2016).
16   Urbach (2015).
17   Engelbracht (2004), pp. 175–202.
18   Engelbracht/Hauser (2013), pp. 90–144.
19   Cf. Atzl/Hess/Schnalke (2005).

consciously or unconsciously, would construct their own biographies in their descriptions.[20] However, processes of self-formation are current of particular interest in the analysis of personal testimonials, of which narrative and biographical interviews are a part.[21] Expert interviews are also essential in the research of nursing history, as only then can nursing routines, which are normally not available in written form, be reconstructed.

This edited volume provides an insight into current research projects in the history of psychiatric nursing in various national contexts and was begun at an international conference, which was held in Stuttgart in October 2015.

The first section "Hospitalisation and Dehospitalisation" is opened with the contribution of Ashild Fause, who researched into the long process of the hospitalisation of the mentally ill in the north of Norway. The specific geographical and demographic conditions meant that home treatment in care foster families was the dominating concept for the therapy of the mentally ill until well into the 20th century. Even in the 1960s and 1970s, only 70 % of the mentally ill were treated in hospitals. Fause analyses the challenges of the family care of psychiatric patients in the 1940s, by investigating care practices and the interactions between caregivers and patients.

By contrast, Sandra Harrisson uses the example of the General Hospital in Ontario, Canada, to investigate how the process of the dehospitalisation of psychiatric care took place in the 1960s. She shows how the activity profile of psychiatric caregivers changed: Their task was now primarily to prepare their patients for an independent life outside the clinic. In so doing, their observations formed the principle basis for treatment plans, which aimed for the fastest possible discharge.

The contribution by Geertje Boschma on the relationship between caregivers, patients and volunteers in the municipal psychiatric institutions in western Canada deals with the process of the dehospitalisation of psychiatric care since the 1970s and the resulting change in the professional self-image of psychiatric caregivers. The anti-authoritarian ideas of the 1960s and 1970s questioned the paternalist and hierarchically-structured relationship between caregivers and patients, gave the patients a voice and required caregivers to reconsider fully their understanding of their profession.

The second section of the book moves the focus to the situation of the patients in the hospital or the clinic and their social surroundings. Jens Gründler has worked on the basis of administration files and patient files of the Scottish asylum Woodilee from the period around 1900 to discover the social conditions under which caregivers worked and what the files have to say about their relationship with the patients. In so doing, Gründler posits the theory that the co-habitation of caregivers and patients in the hospital was usually peaceful, as only few special occurrences are documented in the files. They describe that patients were violent towards caregivers and vice-versa.

---

20 For information on the oral history method in nursing history, cf. Kreutzer (2014), pp. 26–29; Boschma (2008).
21 Cf. Alkemeyer/Budde/Freist (2013).

The circumstance that violent events and complaints by patients were written down causes Gründler to assume that they were regarded as special.

Sylvelyn Hähner-Rombach investigates the "Child Observation Unit" in Innsbruck, Austria, and questions how, from the 1950s, children and young people became patients of this remedial education institution, which was attached to the psychiatric clinic, how they were treated and which consequences their stay had for them and their further life. In addition, she indicates the research potential offered by the comprehensively kept patient files for an interdisciplinary cooperation.

Another perspective on the everyday life of nurses is offered by Sabine Braunschweig in the third section on "Diversity and Deviance" through her contribution on the handling of deviant behaviour by caregivers: She investigates the files on the cancellation of nursing diplomas due to homosexuality, theft and addiction. She is of the opinion that these "deviations" from the "normal" behaviour of the nursing staff allow important insights into the everyday life of nurses. She determines that no intersubjective, comprehensible criteria for the instigation of a procedure to cancel a diploma can be found and suggests that the personal impression that the hospital directors gained of the nurses over time had a decisive role to play.

The fourth section of the book deals with the role of nurses in the introduction and execution of so-called "heroic therapies". In her contribution, Karen Nolte shows the central significance of nursing actions in the execution and evaluation of new forms of electroshock therapies, which were introduced in the 1930s and 1940s in psychiatric treatment at the University Nerve Clinic in Würzburg, Germany. Interestingly, the daily nursing routine only becomes visible in the files with these technically complicated forms of treatment, as nurses were required to document their actions in a detailed and standardised manner.

Foth/Watters/Lange/Connell use their contribution to show the significant role of nurses in "fever treatment" in the Ontario Hospital in Canada. They are of the opinion that the *pyrotherapy* performed by nurses, which consciously took the patients to the brink of death, was primarily used for the social disciplining of uncooperative patients.

The fifth and last section of the book deals with the question of which reforms in the training of nursing personnel in Germany were necessary to be able to reform psychiatry in the sense of the "psychiatric enquête" in 1975. Maike Rotzoll investigates the establishment of the further training of psychiatric caregivers for psychiatry in Heidelberg which had turned into social psychiatry, making it a model for West Germany. From this point onwards, nurses were increasingly expected to have the competences of a social worker. Hierarchies and authoritarian structures were to be dissolved and patients met at eye level.

Christof Beyer analyses the second West German model project on the "further training of psychiatric caregivers" into "sociogogues" at the "Hanover Medical School" in Hanover. He emphasises that the perspective of caregivers on the reform of psychiatry in the 1970s and 1980s has been scarcely investigated. The training programme in Hanover was initially considered to be for nursers in positions of leadership – how this new self-image of psychiatric nurses was received by the grass roots has not yet been investigated.

The aim of this book was not only to sketch the state of international research, but also to point out gaps in research, work upon which would offer new insights into psychiatric nursing. Huge thanks are due to the authors for their substantial contributions.

Bibliography

Alkemeyer, Thomas; Budde, Gunilla; Freist, Dagmar (ed.): Selbst-Bildungen. Soziale und kulturelle Praktiken der Subjektivierung. Bielefeld 2013.

Ankele, Monika: Alltag und Aneignung in Psychiatrie um 1900. Selbstzeugnisse von Frauen aus der Sammlung Prinzhorn. Vienna, Weimar, Cologne 2009.

Atzl, Isabel; Hess, Volker; Schnalke, Thomas (ed.): Zeitzeugen Charité – Arbeitswelten der Psychiatrischen und Nervenklinik 1940–1999. Accompanying book to the exhibition of the Berlin Medical Historical Museum in the Charité, 3rd March to 12th June 2005. Münster 2005.

Blasius, Dirk: Der verwaltete Wahnsinn. Eine Sozialgeschichte des Irrenhauses. Frankfurt/ Main 1980.

Blasius, Dirk: Umgang mit Unheilbaren. Studien zur Sozialgeschichte der Psychiatrie. Bonn 1986.

Borck, Cornelius; Schäfer, Armin (ed.): Das psychiatrische Aufschreibesystem. Paderborn 2015.

Boschma, Geertje: The Rise of Mental Health Nursing. A History of Psychiatric Care in Dutch Asylums, 1890–1920. Amsterdam 2003.

Boschma, Geertje: Oral History Research. In: Lewenson, Sandra B.; Krohn Herrmann, Eleanor (ed.): Capturing Nursing History. A Guide to Historical Methods of Research. New York 2008, pp. 79–98.

Brändli, Sibylle; Lüthi, Barbara; Spuhler, Georg (ed.): Zum Fall machen, zum Fall werden. Wissensproduktion und Patientenerfahrung in Medizin und Psychiatrie des 19. und 20. Jahrhunderts. Frankfurt/Main; New York 2009.

Braunschweig, Sabine: Zwischen Aufsicht und Betreuung. Berufsbildung und Arbeitsalltag der Psychiatriepflege am Beispiel der Basler Heil- und Pflegeanstalt Friedmatt, 1886–1960. Zürich 2013.

Dörner, Klaus: Bürger und Irre: zur Sozialgeschichte und Wissenschaftssoziologie der Psychiatrie. Frankfurt/Main 1984.

Engelbracht, Gerda: Von der Nervenklinik zum Zentralkrankenhaus Bremen-Ost. Bremer Psychiatriegeschichte 1945–1977. Bremen 2004.

Engelbracht, Gerda; Hauser, Andrea: Mitten in Hamburg: die Alsterdorfer Anstalten 1945–1979. Stuttgart 2013.

Faber, Anja: Pflegealltag im stationären Bereich zwischen 1880 und 1930. Stuttgart 2015.

Falkenstein, Dorothee: "Ein guter Wärter ist das vorzüglichste Heilmittel …". Zur Entwicklung der Irrenpflege vom Durchgangs- zum Ausbildungsberuf. Frankfurt/Main 2000.

Fuchs, Petra; Rotzoll, Maike et al. (ed.): "Das Vergessen der Vernichtung ist Teil der Vernichtung selbst". Lebensgeschichten von Opfern der nationalsozialistischen "Euthanasie", Göttingen 2007.

Gründler, Jens: Armut und Wahnsinn. "Arme Irre" und ihre Familien im Spannungsfeld von Psychiatrie und Armenfürsorge in Glasgow, 1875–1921. München 2013.

Höll, Thomas; Schmidt-Michel, Paul-Otto: Irrenpflege im 19. Jahrhundert. Die Wärterfrage in der Diskussion der deutschen Psychiater. Bonn 1989.

Kreutzer, Susanne: Arbeits- und Lebensalltag evangelischer Krankenpflege. Organisation, soziale Praxis und biographische Erfahrungen, 1945–1980. Göttingen 2014.

Ledebur, Sophie: Das Wissen der Anstaltspsychiatrie in der Moderne. Zur Geschichte der Heil- und Pflegeanstalten Am Steinhof in Wien. Vienna; Cologne; Weimar 2015.

Nolte, Karen: Gelebte Hysterie. Erfahrung, Eigensinn und psychiatrische Diskurse im Anstaltsalltag um 1900. Frankfurt/Main, New York 2003.

Nolan, Peter (ed.): A History of Mental Health Nursing. London 1993.

Porter, Roy: The Patient's View: Doing Medical History from below. In: Theory and Society 14 (1985), 2, pp. 175–198.

Urbach, Anna: Das Fallen fixieren. "Epileptikeranstalten" als Wegbereiter einer spezifischen Qualifizierung von psychiatrischen Pflegekräften um 1900. In: Historia Hospitalium 30 (2017).

Urbach, Anna: "Heilsam, förderlich, wirtschaftlich" – Zur Rechtfertigung, Durchführung und Aneignung der Arbeirstherapie in der Landes-Heil- und Pflegeanstalt Uchtspringe 1894–1914. In: Ankele, Monika; Brinkschulte, Eva (ed.): Arbeitsrhythmus und Anstaltsalltag. Arbeit in der Psychiatrie vom frühen 19. Jahrhundert bis in die NS-Zeit, Stuttgart 2015, pp. 71–102.

Hospitalisation and Dehospitalisation

Household Care, Asylums and Nursing Homes.
Facilities and Knowledge in Norwegian Psychiatric Nursing

Åshild Fause

Summary

Legislation on psychiatric care was enacted in Norway in 1848, and since the beginning of the twentieth century three different psychiatric facilities have been used in care and treatment of mentally ill; the publicly supported household care arrangement, psychiatric hospitals named asylums until the 1940'ies in Norway and nursing homes. Despite the fact that the family care system was the most common form of mental health care in Norway until 1940, almost all research has been done on the development in psychiatric institutions. No research has put focus upon the connection between the three levels of care. In Norway, the roots of psychiatric nursing is said to be closely connected to psychiatric institutions. In this article, the intension is, however, to highlight a broader perspective by describing aspects of everyday life and the interaction between the mentally ill and the persons taking care of them in three psychiatric facilities.

The household care facility meant to be taken care of by private people, preferably farming families who received public compensation for having the mentally ill living in their home. The facility was administered by the medical practitioners and by the municipal poor relief, under close inspection and monitoring. The care was, however, a small-scale decentralized system, depended on the presence or proximity of institutions that could be called upon when crisis occurred.

The scene of the investigation is the two northernmost counties in Norway, Troms and Finnmark. Records from the household care facility, written by Medical Practitioners, containing letters from the caretakers, family members and sometimes the mentally ill themselves, telling about everyday life, are analysed together with public statistics in the mental health care arrangements.

At first sight, the daily life activities, interaction and treatment seems to differ a lot between the three facilities. By describing aspects of everyday life and the interaction between mentally ill and those who cared for them, the article investigate which changes occurred and if a line can be drawn from the household care performed by unskilled caretakers to well-educated nurses.

The story of Anna

Anna was born in a small municipality in the county of Troms in 1905. She was a housemaid by profession like many young women in Norway in the first half of the twentieth century. At the age of 25 she attended a religious meeting in her home village and shortly after her behavior and attitude dramatically changed. She could not sleep and continuously cried and bursting out in to tears claiming she was a sinner. Finally a Medical Practitioners (MP) in the area was contacted and asked to come and examine her. According to the MP's record after the home visit, he described Anna as "been strucked by of a seizure of insanity caused by religious brooding".[1] Anna was sent to Rønvik Asylum in Bodø in Nordland County where she stayed for 9 months. Her record tells she was given insulin shock therapy and participated in the daily activities in the asylum, mainly sewing and knitting.[2] Anna slept in wards with 30 other patients. At the time of discharge, she was described as "In progress" and was sent home to her parents. Two years later, "she was hit by another seizure", but this time she was sent to The Nursing Home for mentally ill in Hammerfest in Finnmark County. A few months after, she was placed in household care in the vicinity of Hammerfest. She stayed with her caretakers for nine years, until the deportation of the population in Finnmark and Northern Troms in 1944.[3]

Introduction

The roots of psychiatric nursing in Norway is said to be closely connected to the asylums or the psychiatric hospitals despite the fact that the publicly supported household care was the most common care arrangement in Norway until 1940. The time spent by the mentally ill in hospitals is short in Norway, compared to other countries in Europa.[4] In the period between 1960 and 1975 almost 70 per cent of the mentally ill were taken care of in psychiatric hospitals and public nursing homes. None of the psychiatric hospitals hosted more than 500 patients. But until 1960 the publicly funded household care arrangement was the dominant mode in the Northern part of Norway. Nevertheless, almost all research has had its focus upon the psychiatric institutions.[5] Further, the everyday life experiences of the mentally ill and their household-based caregivers have neither been a main theme in the research field of history of psychiatry, nor in the history of psychiatric nursing. The connection and cooperation between the three levels of care, asylums, nursing homes and household-based care, has almost been of none interest in research.

In this article, my intention is to present a broad perspective on psychiatric nursing and care by describing aspects of everyday life and the interaction between the mentally ill and the persons taking care of them in three types of psychiatric facilities, as the story of Anna tells. Firstly, I will focus on the pub-

---

1 Regional State Archive in Tromsø (RSAT): Fylkesmannen i Troms, Sinnssyke i forpleining (FFT) (County Governor in Troms, Records of mentally ill), box 2839.
2 RSAT, FFT, box 2839.
3 Norway was occupied by Germany in 1940–1945 and from February 1942 the Government was led by Nazi German dictatorship. As a part of the withdrawal from the Litza front on the Kola Peninsula, the Germans effectuated the scorched earth strategy in October 1944, and more than 50,000 inhabitants from the county of Finnmark and from the northern part of the county of Troms were deported southwards. Among them were 150 mentally ill. For further reading see Fause (2015).
4 Pedersen (2002), p. 188.
5 Fause (2007), pp. 15–16.

licly supported and supervised household care arrangement, conducted by unskilled caretakers; secondly I will deal with nurses and attendants in an asylum or psychiatric hospital and a nursing home.

The scene of the investigation is the two northernmost counties in Norway, Troms and Finnmark. Finnmark is by area the largest county in Norway, as big as Denmark. The population numbered approximately 56.000 inhabitants in 1940 while there was a total of approximately 350.000 in the Northern region.[6] The natural environment is generous in the sense that the sea provides food and employment, but the climate is harsh, and it is hard to succeed with extensive farming. Troms is a county located south of Finnmark, with a population twice as large. Troms was in the 1940s mainly populated by farmer-fishermen living on small farms along the coastline and in the fjords. An underlying hypothesis in this article is that everyday life of the rural type, with its multitude of tasks, seasons, cooperation and interaction has been and still is an important factor on the way to recover and gain strength for people with mental problems.

At first sight, everyday activities, interaction, care and treatment seems to differ a lot between the three different psychiatric facilities. In this article I ask if there are any connections and similarities between nursing and care as it developed in the three arrangements? Where there any differences in the way the patients were looked upon by the staff and caretakers in the three psychiatric facilities? Did the everyday activities and the interaction between patients and the persons taking care of them differ within the three facilities?

Sources used

This is an empirical study based upon different sources. *Case records* written by Medical Practitioners' (MP) in Northern Norway have been the most important sources. To become registered as mentally ill in Norway, the person involved were examined by a MP, who kept records. In pre-war Norway the mentally ill often went in and out of the mentally health care system, just as they do today, and every time new remarks were made in the records. In some cases one can follow a person on his or hers way through the mentally health care system for 30 to 40 years. In these records you also find letters from the caretakers, neighbors, and family members and in some few cases, also letters written by the mentally ill themselves. It is obvious that these are mostly letters of complaints, but by contextualizing these letters, it is also possible to interpret how the patients thought about the treatment and care they were offered. In addition to records the MP's also made *annual reports on the health condition* of the population in their region. These reports give an overview not only of the health conditions, but also living conditions in general. Together with *Annual Statistics from the Psychiatric Hospitals* and *Statistics of the Publicly*

---

6   Folkemengdens Bevegelser (Cencus) (1946).

financed Family Care Arrangement in Norway, archives from a nursing home and a psychiatric hospital in Northern Norway have been used to provide additional insight to the field studied. In order to illustrate, illuminate or concretize the sources used, and bring forth detailed and thorough knowledge, interviews with 5 persons raised with mentally in their households, are conducted.[7] The purpose was to provide a more detailed picture of how the mentally ill were perceived and taken care of by others in the household care arrangement.

The publicly supported household care[8]

Being offered household care meant to be taken care of by private people, preferably in farming – fishery households. The family received public compensation for having the mentally ill living in their home. Based on a contract signed by representatives of the county, the caregiver and the municipal authority, the responsibilities of the caregiver, the economic compensation granted and the care period, which was normally one year, were defined. The contract could be prolonged, but also terminated if conditions were not met to satisfaction.

Historians describe the Norwegian household as *an arena where you actually live your everyday life*.[9] The concept of "household" is not synonymous with that of family; as it was a production unit, often including also non-family members and (unmarried) relatives. Even if the household structure changed gradually during the period, by becoming more like a modern family, its main features were yet the same. Having lodgers who also participated in meals and spent time with the other family members was not unusual. Elderly people without relatives in the communities were taken care of in the households on behalf of the local poverty board.

In Northern Norway, the combination of production for subsistence and for the market lasted longer than in other parts of Norway.[10] Throughout the 20th century there was a gradual change in the way of living but this change took place later than in other parts of the country. Even if there were technological changes within farming and fisheries, and there was a growth in manufacturing industries, the farming-fisheries household survived this first modernizing process.[11] The housewife ran the farm and managed the household, in periods while the male family members participated in seasonal fisheries away from home. Meanwhile not all households managed to produce and sell enough goods to take care of their members. These households were given

7   Slettan (1994) p. 124; Kjelstadli (1999) p. 193.
8   This chapter is based upon Fause (2007), chapter 6.
9   Balsvik (1991) p. 639.
10   Elstad (1991), p. 593.
11   Bjørklund et al. (1984).

poverty support.[12] Money was in short supply for the greater part of the population, and as more fabricated commodities became available, income from wage labour outside the household was needed to be able to buy them.

According to the contract, the caregiver was responsible for the support of the mentally ill and for the agreed upon sum, he or she was obliged to provide the mentally ill person with proper clothes and food, a good and heated bedroom, a bed with bed linen, outdoor activities and suitable work. The contract obliged the caregiver to monitor the activities of the mentally ill to try to prevent him or her from wandering around the neighbourhood and act in such a way as to put themselves or others in danger. If a person placed in the household care tried to escape, the caregiver was obliged to cover the costs incurred by bringing the mentally ill person back to the household.

The MP's reported annually, on the basis of home visits, how the household care functioned for the mentally ill, and the reports were compiled and transmitted to the medical authorities at the regional and national level. Together with reports from the hospitals and nursing homes, these reports formed the basis for statistics on mental health care. The majority of the individuals registered as mentally ill were kept in household care in the patient's own municipality or county. This care system was extremely small-scale and decentralized. As the care arrangement developed in Northern Norway, there was as a general rule no more than one, and only in a few cases two, mentally ill in each caretaking household. This arrangement was quite different from the care model developing in other regions of Norway; often mentioned as "colonies" of 10 up to 20 mentally ill in each colony.[13]

From the records we learn that the household based system did not operate on its own, with the district MP as the sole provider of monitoring and expert knowledge. The system depended on the presence of, or the proximity of institutions that could be called upon when the need for full-time care or critical situations occurred. To meet this demand, institutions like ordinary hospitals, but also police custody and jails provided arrangements to take care of the mentally ill in situations of emergency, i.e. when the private care was unable to cope with problematic incidents. Without these institutions as a "back-up" the household based care system hardly would have become consolidated as the dominant form of care in the counties in Northern Norway. The household based care system was exposed to criticism, especially by the psychiatrists and physicians in the psychiatric hospitals, but since the arrangements seemed to function and due to the lack of public funding for an additional psychiatric hospital in Northern Norway, the system was maintained, and was in fact as the dominant form of care over a century until Åsgård Psychiatric Hospital opened in Troms County, in 1961.

The Norwegian household cannot be seen as "a private place"; in the sense of a closed sphere, as families or family based households are thought of nowadays. The household was not an arena for protected privacy, but rather a

---

12   Andresen (1994), p. 360.
13   Bøe (1993); Bauer (1995) and Lia (2003).

semi-public place with members participating in farm work, housework, maintenance, care and nursing. Farming was especially important, and the household was both a place to live and to work. The tasks varied with the seasons, some were simple use of labour manual work and other tasks were complex and based on knowledge and special skills. Household members would typically cooperate in these different tasks. There was always a lot of work that had to be done. The caretaker was responsible for the mentally ill for 24 hours; it was a day and night responsibility. The concept of household therefore make it possible to understand the care outside the hospitals since it presupposes a focus on how the mentally ill were integrated in everyday life practices, including how bodily needs and nuisances were handled.

For the mentally ill, who according to the MP's, was in need of professional psychiatric treatment, transportation to the psychiatric hospitals in the south was arranged, but even the distance within the region, from Eastern Finnmark to Bodø could be more than 1200 kilometres.

Rønvik State Asylum in Bodø

While somatic medicine made great success at the beginning of the 20th Century, pessimism increased within psychiatric institutions.[14] Results from treatments failed to appear and so-called chronic patients filled up the institutions. The difficulties of getting qualified attendants increased and the public supported family care arrangements, were criticized. It was in this period the Rønvik Asylum opened in Bodø.

The main aim behind establishing asylums in Norway was to improve the conditions for the mentally ill. Norwegian psychiatrists expressed the asylum's main task as to represent high moral standards, sympathy and humanity, but also modernization and progress.[15] The hospitalization was a "moral" treatment, but also prevention against suicide and violence. The asylum provided a calm and regular life, with structure and cleanliness, where the patients could embody new habits that put them in interaction with the environment, work was said to restore health, and the asylum area included (by North Norwegian standards) a large scale farming enterprise. Due to the demand to the asylum of being self-sufficient, the patients' labor was of great importance; and was named work therapy.

By 1940 Rønvik Asylum had a capacity of 264 beds and 471 inpatients.[16] Some wards could provide up to 30 beds. The so-called "subdued treatment" consisting of bed resting and prolonged baths was common until 1920. From 1920 optimism spread in Norwegian psychiatry as the number of asylum beds increased and new treatments were introduced. Over the next decades to come the asylums in Norway were transformed into medical institutions using

14   Ludvigsen (1998), p. 54.
15   Sandmo (2005), p. 53.
16   Sinnssykehusenes virksomhet (1940–1945).

treatments like shock therapies, surgery and medication; these were forms of treatment underlining the somatic character of mental disorders.[17] The new methods were soon implemented at Rønvik Asylum. In this situation educated nurses were demanded. But parallel to the somatic turn, work therapy was maintained and formed part of the everyday life in the psychiatric institutions.

The Nursing Home in Hammerfest

The nursing home for mentally ill in Hammerfest opened in 1930 and was the first public institution of a considerable scope dedicated to the care of the mentally ill in Troms and Finnmark.[18] It was established to care for mentally ill patients regarded as incurable, with no expectations of a return to normality. The home had a capacity of 56 beds, but more than 100 patients lived there at the time of its closure in 1942. It was the biggest nursing home for mentally ill in Norway at the time.[19] The MP's of Hammerfest municipality was the manager and the Betanien Methodist nursing school in Oslo recruited trained nurses to run it. The Hammerfest Nursing Home also trained nurses and attendants. This happened in the 1930s, at a time of crisis in both public and private sector economies. The lack of beds at the psychiatric hospitals in Norway had become precarious during the 1920s and consequently it was hard for the MP's to have a patient sent to Rønvik Asylum for treatment and care. In addition, it was difficult to find caretakers, due to the low number of farming households in the fishery and reindeer herding-dominated Finnmark County. The mentally ill were therefore mostly placed in household care in Troms and Nordland, and the costs for this care were high. The nursing home was soon filled up with patients from Finnmark, Troms and even from the county of Nordland where Rønvik Asylum was situated. During the time period of the institutions' existence, patients from Rønvik Asylum and mentally ill living in household care in Nordland also moved back to Finnmark; at first to the nursing home in Hammerfest, but soon after to caretakers in the Hammerfest area. Due to the lack of paid employment in the 1930s, the nursing home had no problems in recruiting household caretakers (mostly non-farm households in this case). This situation changed dramatically during wartime. Since the Germans could offer paid labour, some caretakers cancelled their contracts and found working for the Germans much more convenient than taking care of the mentally ill inside their houses.

The nursing home functioned until 1942, when the Germans requisitioned the home for military purposes and by 1944 the patients were evacuated together with the population, most of them to asylums in the south. Due

17　Fause (2013), pp. 111–113.
18　Fause (2009), p. 94.
19　Fause (2009), p. 94.

to the Scorched Earth tactics practiced by the German occupants, almost every building in Finnmark and Northern Troms, were put on fire.[20]

What changes occurred in the care between the three facilities?

The three facilities were all based upon a 24 hours care, but the level of structure and formalization differed. In the following, 6 factors will be highlighted while asking what are the connections and similarities between nursing and care as it developed within the three types? Did the everyday activities and the interaction between patients and the persons taking care of them change when unskilled caretakers were replaced by educated nurses? Where there any differences in the way the patients were looked upon in the three psychiatric facilities?

The need of education in psychiatric care

During the years when farming and participating in everyday activities was a central part of the asylum's treatment, it was easy to get attendants with experience and competence from traditional handicraft – or agricultural trades.[21] After being established as a specialty in medicine in late 1890's in Norway, the psychiatrists raised the question if not caring for mentally ill demanded peculiar knowledge and skills and the need for a special training in psychiatric care was launched. Doctor J. Heinrichs argued that the employees needed to know more than how to prevent patients to harm themselves and to care for their physical needs. The best way to learn how to care for the mentally ill was by combining work in the wards with theoretical knowledge. The attendants were lectured in observing signs and symptoms on mentally diseases in order to apply the pertinent psychiatric treatments.[22]

In 1900 the first program in nursing was launched for staff at Gaustad Asylum.[23] The term "guardian" simultaneously was changed to attendant and nurse. That same year the staff organized their own attendant associations and joined the Norwegian Trade Union Confederation (LO). Rønvik Asylum established course lasting 18 hours in 1913.[24] Soon after the course expanded to a one year course and 10 male attendants and female nurses got their exams every year.[25] However, we do not know much about how the courses were organized. According to the asylum regulation, a consultant gave lectures together with the head nurse.

20 Fause (2015).
21 Borgan/Søraa (1972), p. 100.
22 Heinrich (1914), p. 71.
23 Saastad (1995), p. 93.
24 Borgan/Søraa (1972), p. 100; Fygle (2002), p. 82.
25 Fygle (2002), p. 82.

During the 1930'es all Norwegian asylums employed trained female nurses at the male wards and the training courses were expanded to a two years program.[26] The question was whether the competence should be based upon the 3 years program in nursing or should Norway develop an independent school program in psychiatric nursing like it was in Great Britain, The Netherlands, Finland, etc. The Norwegian Nurse Association considered that psychiatric nursing was only one of several fields of interests in nursing and argued that psychiatric nursing should become a specialty in nursing based on the 3 year program.[27]

The Act of Nursing of 1948 had provided nurses with 3-years nursing program the opportunity to apply for certification as registered nurse. In the future public approval could only be achieved by completing the 3-years nursing program. The problem was temporarily that the nurse organization, from its establishment in 1912, was a federation reserved for women only. Men could not apply for admission to nursing schools, but could be admitted as a student at the Norwegian Deacon Home 1890.[28] The law was therefore a compromise with special adaptations for male attendants with long experience in psychiatric hospitals. Authorized nurses could take transition to midwifery schools and psychiatric nursing schools after 2 years and 4 months. The Act of Nursing in 1948 gave male attendants access to apply for admission to the nursing educations and become members of the association. Some of the attendants did, but most of them remained working as nurse assistants.

Comparing the household care arrangement with the institutions, the only requirement the authorities demanded from the caretakers, was that they themselves did not receive poor relief support. Both the poverty boards in each municipality and the MP's were aware of the impact of financial support on the caretakers' economic situation. The financial contribution was a welcomed addition to the economy in the households. They also knew for certain that some applied to care for the mentally ill just for the money. In the period analyzed, it had come to the MP's and local poverty board's knowledge, which of the caretakers was trustworthy and reliable in handling mentally ill persons. Both regional and State authorities emphasized the caretakers' ability to handle unexpected situations that could occur in the households like anxiety and disruptive behavior, as well as the ability to offer the mentally ill suitable labor etc. Some caretaker milieus emerged, and were frequently called upon. This was particularly the case in some municipalities in Nordland County like Steigen and Misvær.[29] In these communities the inhabitants for decades had a relatively high number of mentally ill in care proportional to the population. But also communities in the counties of Buskerud and Akershus County in the Southern part of Norway, were considered to be suitable for caring outside

26 Leikvam (1935), p. 16.
27 Hvalvik (2005), p. 280.
28 Stave (1990).
29 Fause (2007), p. 168.

the asylum. During the 1930s some district MP's in northern Norway argued that all homes were not suited to take care of mentally ill, and particularly nurses residing in rural areas were preferred as caretakers.[30]

In the asylum and nursing homes knowledge had become specialized. The treatment were implemented by specialist telling the attendants and nurses how to behave and what to do. The staff observed the patients' behavior and reported to the head nurse, who also gave orders. Observation became more important than communication and relationships.

Considering the mentally ill as sick

The attendants and nurses at Rønvik Asylum and Hammerfest Nursing Home were according to the regulations not allowed to use words and phrases such as "mad", "crazy", "silly" or "frivolous" about the mentally ill.[31] The staff could thus no longer use everyday language expressions in their chat and conversation with the patients, but had to change their language. The management exhorted employees to try to avoid conflict and use of the "heavy hand" in dealing with the sick. None of the staff had the authority to compel the sick, but they could turn to their immediate supervisor if the use of force was required. Mistreatment of patients would result in immediate dismissal. The patients could not be isolated without the head nurse's permission. If so happened, the incident immediately would be reported to the managers. Simultaneous, the regulations emphasized, if possible, the impact of accommodate any reasonable request from the patients. Furthermore, the staff should also act with vigilance and attention when relating to patients. It was particularly important to ensure that patients did not harm other patients or themselves or destroyed or damaged the institution's inventory. The staff was trained to treat the mentally ill with patience and without violence. Any hint of revenge against the patient's behavior, had to be avoided, likewise to express great familiarity.

The staff was further strongly advised to prevent outbursts of emotions among the patients. Religious conversations with patients were strictly forbidden and to receive gifts or their next to kin were not allowed. The patients had no entrance to the staff's bed rooms. Such guidelines led to a distance between the patients and those who cared of them. In addition, the patients' ailments and problems became highly visible in everyday life when those who nursed them also should observe and record their behavior and interaction.

This differed from the practices of the household care outside the institution. Here the mentally ill were integrated in the household and was entrusted with responsibilities as the following example tells. A man, who grew up with a mentally ill in his home in a municipality in Troms, said he and his two

30   Fause (2007), p. 170.
31   Regulations of Rønvik Asylum of 1902, Regulation of the Nursing Home for Mentally Ill in Hammerfest of (1930).

brothers for several years slept in the same bedroom as the mentally ill.[32] It was perceived safe for the children. "When Martin", as the man was named, "followed us to the outdoor bathroom in the evenings, we never felt anxious. He was strong and always helpful". The example tells us that the mentally ill in some cases were seen as family member and was entrusted with responsibilities to the children.

The importance of labor

In all three facilities participation in daily activities was of great importance but the outcome of the work effort differed. From the opening of Gaustad State Asylum in 1855, labor was said to have a healing effect on the mentally ill.[33] Contact with animals and soil would help to balance the split mind and it was a widespread belief that the best cure for insomnia, was outdoor activities. In the household care the caretaker, according to the contract, was responsible to provide labor for the mentally ill and the household work offered a wide range of tasks of varying difficulties.[34] Male and female patients participated in different tasks assigned on ability and skills. Women were set to card, spin, knit and sew, while men participated in labor on the farm or in the fisheries. Wood needed to be cut, cleaved, stacked and carried into the house and the same with water since running water was uncommon in the households. In some records, the MP often wrote that the work ability of some female was at a minimum, but at least they were able to knit. Both men and women were set to perform labor they were used to carry out from childhood. The most simple farm – and household work – either indoors or outdoors, was crucial for both the household and the mentally ill. Taking part in the everyday tasks throughout the day in the household helped to maintain a structure in the daily life for the mentally ill.

The following story describes the impact everyday tasks had for the running of the household.[35] A man who was in private family care was responsible for carrying wood and water into the house. At one occasion the housewife in the family asked him to go and get more firewood. The man instead wanted a cup of coffee but was told to fetch the wood first. This made the man annoyed at the housewife and without saying a word; he carried some wood that already was lying in the wood box, out to the woodshed. Unless he got coffee, he refused to obey the housewife's request. End of the story was that the housewife had to put on the coffee pot and serve the man a cup of coffee before he brought in the wood. The man's work was of major importance to running the household, but the housewife also knew from experience that if

32 Informant no 2.
33 Evensen (1908), p. 995.
34 Fause (2007), p. 151.
35 Informant no 2.

the mentally ill's temper was trigged, his mood would change rapidly, and make a lot of challenges for the household's members.

The contributions were assessed and determined by the degree of effort and benefit to the household. If a male mentally ill could help with farm work or fishing, the financial contribution were set less than if the person required more supervision and caused more trouble in the household. To receive an annual cash grant was a significant contribution to the economy of the household. The contribution was not so much that a family could live on it, but it gave cash income, which was scarce among the population in the relevant period. Individuals were given a more spacious economy by the cash contribution and the authorities could be assured that the insane were taken care of – in one way or another. Thus the state saved money, since asylum catering was far more expensive.

It is not evident claiming that household care was more beneficial for the mentally ill as a general rule, compared to hospitalization, but if the caretaker and the household members acted as "good and wise people", the arrangement might be the best solution for the person.

Patient work was also assessed in nursing homes and asylum. Staff should encourage patients to participate in the activities the nursing home and care center could offer. Patients were assigned duties by the management's judgment. All work should as a rule be performed under the supervision of a nurse or an attendant, unless the manager saw it otherwise. The patient effort was documented in annual reports of the nursing homes and asylum. Both the manager of Rønvik Asylum and the manager of Hammerfest Nursing Home underlined that it was significant for both the patients' well-being and health, but also for economic purposes, that patients participated in the work. The institutions depended on the patient's efforts to keep the budget.

Both Rønvik Asylum and the Hammerfest nursing home had separate wards for male and female patients. In the male wards the patients crafted, painted and performed various maintenance works. While farm work was important at Rønvik Asylum, the patients at the nursing home in Hammerfest leveled gravel paths outside the buildings. At both institutions the patients and the staff established parks and gardens in the summertime, while basketry and bookbinding were indoors activities during wintertime. In the 1940s encouragement money was introduced to the patients who participated in the daily activities.

By comparing the work carried out in the institutions and in the household care, there are similarities but also some differences. The work performed by the patients was needed in both types of facilities and the tasks of the institutions might be seen as a continuation of the tasks traditionally performed in the households.

Taking part in activities in work rooms, however, was modeled after the industry and changed both work function and the purpose itself. From being a necessary part of the work in the household, the work was now also said to be an essential part of daily therapy; referred to as occupational therapy. Patients in nursing homes and in the asylum performed their duties and at regular intervals during the day and working hours were as their day of leisure, structured according to the clock. In household care the tasks followed a day, a week or a year cycle. In the household there were not a marked difference between working hours and leisure time.[36] The concept of time was oriented towards tasks, cyclic and followed the rhythm of the day and the year, not the time of the clock. The members of the household participated in tasks at different times of the day, and the distinction between work and leisure was diffuse, in opposition to the institutions where both patients and staff had a clear separation between working hours and leisure time.

From individual responsibility to hierarchically assignment

In the household care the mentally ill were allowed to walk around in the surroundings as he or she would unless extra guarding was required. Many stayed in the same household for years and became familiar with the people in the neighborhood. The caretaker was according to the contract, responsible if the mentally ill ran off and had to finance the costs for bringing the person home. It was not unusual that some roamed in local surroundings in periods before being halted and transported back to the household. In many villages the inhabitants established "teams of guards" (Norwegian: "vaktlag") of men who could be called upon to keep watch over the mentally ill when needed. Not only the single household, but the rural community was in many ways involved in the care by handling or managing deviant behaviour and aggression by the insane. This led the mentally ill into a broad contact with inhabitants in the surrounding areas and participation in various activities in the local communities.

Being a caretaker was challenging and demanding in many ways. Although the care arrangement was contractual, the daily exercise was entrusted to the caretaker to consider how to handle the different situations. It was not uncommon to resort to coax, coffee and tobacco in order to avoid conflicts. The relationship between the caretaker and the mentally ill was of great significance for the interaction between them. Proponents of the household care, argued that a caretaker also being a farmer, house wife or craftsman: "put more effort, power and interest in the labor because the outcome of the mentally ill's work is a part of the income of the household". It would not be the same in the institutions where the staff was only wage earners. A caretaker had a personal interest in keeping the mentally ill in a good mood, and the use of small talk, rewards, praise, etc. was useful techniques to get the work done. If the relationship between the caretaker and mentally ill was characterized only by a strict tone, that person would refuse to work.

A woman being born and raised in a family with a mentally ill in care in a small community in Finnmark, told that her father and the mentally ill al-

---

36   Elstad (1991), p. 593.

ways worked together whether it was fishing or farm work.[37] They also dressed in the same kind of clothes and at long distances it was hard to tell them apart. When her father was away, the man went to his room and lay down on the bed until her father returned home. The man would not deal with anyone in the house but the father.

In the institutions the manager was responsible for the treatment. In his absence the responsibility was delegated to the head nurse who distributed tasks and activities to the staff. Activities linked to treatment and care followed guidelines determined by the chief physicians. Simultaneously work was carried out meticulously, reliably and securely. If something unforeseen happened in the follow-up of patients, employees had to immediately notify the sister who reported to the superintendent. The management decided who was allowed to attend the prayer, outage, work and participation in various activities.

The institutions had a daily rhythm that everyone had to follow. The patients were awakened and went to bed at regular times. The employees worked for a fixed hours. Apart from the male attendants who had family, the female staff lived their lives at the institution. The staff could not come and leave without the permission or have visitors. Because they lived inside the institution's area, there was a vague distinction between work and leisure time, just like as it was for the caretakers in the households. But employees of institutions were subject to clock time and working long hours and little free time. They could not come and go as they would when they had leisure time. The management team expected that the staff were available. Employees were required to follow the guidelines for the daily follow-up of patients and discipline was evident in the requirements and expectations of both staff and patients. The leaders and especially the head nurse had a central role in the education of the staff. Regulations required that staff were obedient, submissive and dutiful towards superiors. At the same time, there were clear expectations for staff to show patients attention and be patient. They were also instilled to protect the sick and simultaneously strengthen the nursing home's reputation.

In an article in a Medical Periodical in 1935, a physician at Rønvik Asylum, criticized what he called the hard and almost inhuman working conditions the staff had in the asylum; especially the educated nurses[38]. He mentioned in particular the strict discipline, the regulations, the long working days, lack of leisure time and emphasized especially what negative effects such working conditions might have the care of the patients. From a medical point of view he argued that improvements in employees' working and pay conditions would benefit the patients. He stressed the impact of being unionized and thus to be positioned to demand better working conditions.

---

37   Informant no 2.
38   Leikvam (1935).

Confidentiality

In nursing homes and asylums the staff was responsible for strict monitoring of the patients.[39] Both Rønvik Asylum and Hammerfest Nursing Home were surrounded by tall fences within which the patients were allowed to move freely. The attendants and nurses were imposed strict silence about what they experienced in the daily work and not, under any circumstances, to tell anyone about what happened behind the fences. The regulations and guidelines may be compared with the regimentation of staff and patients, in line with Michel Foucault's analysis of discipline in psychiatric institutions more than a hundred years earlier.[40]

The requirements for the staff followed the same rules and guidelines for both asylum and other hospital during this time.[41] Usually patients were not allowed to leave the hospitals without seeking permission and visitors had to show access cards to enter a hospital.

Regulatory management was not entrenched and the manager of the nursing home was keen to find solutions as the following example shows. A woman, with several stays at Rønvik Asylum, was admitted to the nursing home.[42] A few weeks after admission, it was noted that the woman was pregnant. According to the manager, the pregnancy had so far had a positive impact on the woman, and he decided that she would carry the pregnancy and keep the baby after birth. She was therefore placed in household care in an appropriately well suited care few weeks after birth.

A tension between control and humanism

Even before the turn of the century caring for mentally ill was said to be an important field of nursing. Deaconess Rikke Nissen states in her textbook in 1877:

> To recover from mental illness, demands a calm and regular life style combined with an appropriate diversion between rest and activity. Fresh air is as important as a good night sleep is. His sleep must not be disturbed when needed, but staying in bed all day long is as worse as insomnia.[43]

Rikke Nissen wrote the textbook into the tradition of the moral treatment and emphasized that human dignity is not only being decided in relation to fellow human beings, but also in relation to the environment, housing and how we interact with each other and the daily chores.[44] Here we find a parallel to Florence Nightingale showing how nursing by providing circadian rhythms,

39   Fygle (2002), pp. 61–63.
40   Foucault (2001), pp. 127–128.
41   Elstad (2006), p. 367.
42   RSAT, FFT, box 2865 (1909–1943).
43   Nissen 1877 (2000), p. 74.
44   Nissen 1877(2000), p. 75.

fresh air, food, customizable amount of rest and activity, place the body into such a state that nature's own healing powers can act on it.[45] By cultivate the nurses to "patience, love, wisdom and courteous" in the relationship with the patient while conducting the doctor's orders and the guidelines, Nissen suggest an ambiguity between control versus humanism.

Contemporary literary texts may provide knowledge about people's daily experience of his day reality.[46] The Norwegian author Amalie Skram gives in her novels "Professor Hieronimus" and "In Sct. Jørgen" an insight into the conditions in psychiatric institutions at the end of the 1900s and refers to tensions between coercion, power and control against a humanistic attitude. In describing the staff as both guardians and caring nurses, Skram highlights a duality in the nurses demeanor as she describes the nurses as "pale rays on a dark and ice frozen winter".[47] The following statements describes a nurse who has hurt his patient and which expresses it: "Dear Little Lady, we all do wish you the best" or "I feel sorry for you Mrs. Kant, and wish you so well".[48] The nurse Ms Hansen tells Mrs. Kant to be calm and encouraged her to win the professor's confidence since undesirable behavior within the psychiatric institution may be interpreted as a serious mental disease. "The professor does well with those he likes", said Ms. Hansen.[49]

On one hand, the nurses acted as the physician's good assistants due to their rank as subordinated to them in the asylum hierarchy, but meanwhile they also conducted confidentiality and humanized the stay and treatment for patients. It is this tension the Norwegian nurse and philosopher Kari Martinsen stresses as the ambiguous in the moral treatment.[50] By setting limits and exercise control in a dignified way, the treatment becomes a protection against "the limitless". In the moral treatment tradition both disciplinary and compelling actions was a challenge that the employees had to live with.

According to Karin Neuman-Rahn who worked for decades as a psychiatric nurse in Finland from the 1920s, the nurse's main task was to win the patient's trust and confidence.[51] During the psychiatrist's and physician's invasive examinations and treatment, the nurses' main responsibility was to protect the patients from pain and offense.[52] As we see it is a line from Rikke Nissen in the 1870s arguing that nursing mentally ill requires special skills and appropriateness at a time when psychiatric treatment became more intrusive.[53]

Whether the care was performed in family care or in psychiatric institutions, the conduct was in a field of tension between taking care of and exercise control over the person. In Jenny Björkmanns study of coercion in Swedish

45   Nightingale (1997), p. 32.
46   Kjelstadli (2005), p. 165.
47   Skram: Professor (1977), p. 88.
48   Skram: Professor (1977), p. 60.
49   Skram: På (1977), p. 90.
50   Martinsen (2001), p. 183.
51   Neuman-Rahn (1924).
52   Neuman-Rahn (1924).
53   Mathialainen (1997).

legislation for the period 1850–1970 she highlights the conceptual pair "caring" and "controlling" as ever present in psychiatric treatment.[54] "Caring" means to care for someone; to provide, look after or to protect the other from an inhuman setting, while "controlling" means to set limits, stick, watching over, etc. She claims however that it is not certain that coercion, control, normalization and discipline are opposites of a good, humane and civilized practice.

Being together with the mentally ill in everyday life, both within the institution or in household care, the care was often challenging. Giving competent praise and encouragement when needed and scolding and reproof on other occasions, was the way life unfolded in both places. Caring for mentally ill meant both a humanistic attitude, but also control. Sometimes the mentally ill required a larger degree of control than the household could offer. In these cases the mentally ill were moved to a facility offering a stricter and higher level of control, like a ward in Rønvik Asylum. In other occasions the MP's found the household care to be unsatisfactory due to an excessive degree of control and insufficient safeguarding. It was not uncommon that employees of the asylum were dismissed because of incidents of coercion against patients. Balancing between "take care of" and "to control" was something the nurses and attendants were aware of and encountered many times a day, but still it was hard to find the balance.

Closing remarks

Everyday life and work had an important impact in both the psychiatric institutions and in the household care. Work was considered being of great importance for individual's mental state, while regarded as a necessary contribution to the financial situation of the household and to the institutions.

In family care the mentally ill occasionally caused problems and the caretaker and the rest of the family had to deal with the situations. In institutions the staff was trained to deal with the mentally ill as sick and as different from themselves. A specialized psychiatric knowledge became a necessity. This led to a professionalization of the field and within the institutions the staff became employees in a hierarchy where the manager and the head nurse defined the rules and developed guidelines.

The relationship between the mentally ill and the staff changed within the institutions. Regarding the patients as sick, made their many problems, bothers and suffering visible as well as their strange behavior. In this article, I have shown that the three types of handling the mentally ill did not operate in separate spheres, but were rather well integrated, as patients have been found to move between the types, based on professional judgements of what would be the best place for the individual patient. As for differences and similarities

54   Bjørkmann(2001), p. 25.

in everyday life practices, the difference between the daily rhythm of the household life and that of the asylum is significant. The knowledge and practices of the educated nurses however, seem to mitigate the effects of what could be characterized as inhuman structures of the fenced-in institution.

Bibliography

Archival sources

National Archive in Norway (NA)

Medisinalinnberetninger for Finnmark, Troms og Nordland (Annual Reports from the County Medical Officer of Finnmark, Troms and Nordland).
Sosialdepartementet, Kontoret for psykiatri, H4 (Ministry of Social Affairs, Office of Psychiatry H4).
Flyktninge- og fangedirektoratet, Direktoratets distriktskontorer med forløpere (Directorate of Refuges and Prisoners of War, Districts Offices).

Regional State Archive in Tromsø (RSAT)

Fylkesmannen i Troms, Sinnssyke i forpleining (County Governor in Troms, Records of Mentally Ill).
Fylkesmannen i Finnmark (County Governor in Finnmark).
Fylkeslegen i Troms (Chief County Medical Officer in Troms).
Fylkeslegen i Finnmark (Chief County Medical Officer in Finnmark).

Private archive Åshild Fause

Interview no 1: Female, born in Finnmark County, Interview made the author, May 15, 2006.
Interview no 2: Male, born in Troms County, Interview made by the author, May 23, 2005.

Printed Sources

Folkemengdens bevegelser 1946 (Census 1946).
Forarbeid for Lov om Psykisk Helsevern, 1956 (Preparation of Act of Mental Health Care, 1956).
Forhandlingsprotokoller for Finnmark Fylke (FFF), Sinnssykeberetninger, 1900–1950 (Negotiation protocols County Council of Finnmark, Annual Reports of Mentally Ill).
Forhandlingsprotokoller for Troms Fylke (FFT), Sinnssykeberetninger, 1900–1950 (Negotiation protocols County Council of Troms, Annual Reports of Mentally Ill).
Sinnssykeasylenes virksomhet / Sinnssykehusenes virksomhet (1873–1950) (Annual Statistics from Norwegian asylums / Psychiatric Hospitals 1873–1950).

Secondary research literature

Andresen, Astri: Handelsfolk og fiskerbønder. Tromsø gjennom 10 000 år. Bind 2. Tromsø 1994.

Balsvik, Randi R.: "Kvinner i nordnorske kystsamfunn". In: Historisk Tidsskrift 4 (1991), pp. 335–355.

Bauer, Tom J.: Åtte gærninger og to vettu'e. Privatforpleining av sinnssyke i Nes på Romerike 1900–1961. Årnes 1995.

Borgan, Valborg og Gerd Søraa: Rotvoll 1872–1972: Fra asyl for sinnssyke til psykiatriske sykehus. Trondheim 1972.

Bjørklund, Ivar, Einar Arne Drivenes og Siri Gerrard (1984): "På vei til det moderne. Om jordbruk, fiske, reindrift og industri 1890–1990". In: Einar Arne Drivenes, Marit Hauan og Helge A. Wold : Nordnorsk kulturhistorie. Det gjenstridige landet. Oslo 1984. pp. 104–122.

Bjørkmann, Jenny: Vård för samhällets bäste. Debatten om tvångsvård i svensk lagstifting 1850–1970. Uppsala 2001.

Bøe, Jon B.: De utsatte. Psykiatriske pasienter i privatpleie på Jæren 1950–197. Oslo 1993.

Elstad, Å.: "Mentalitet og økonomi – Nord-Noreg 1750–1950". In: Historisk Tidsskrift 4 (1991), pp. 586–603.

Evensen, Hans: Grunntrekkene i det norske sindsygevæsens udvikling i de sidste 100 år. In: Tidsskrift for Den Norske Lægeforening 2 (1905), pp. 22–29.

Fause, Åshild: "Forpleiningen tilfredsstillende. Prisen ligesaa". Sinnssykeomsorgen i Troms og Finnmark 1891–1940. Phd-avhandling i helsevitenskap, Universitetet i Tromsø 2007.

Fause, Åshild: The Nursing Home for Mentally Ill in Hammerfest, 1930–1942. In: Andresen, A. et al. (ed.): Healthcare Systems and Medical Institutions. Oslo 2009. pp. 94–102.

Fause, Åshild: Framveksten av psykiske helsetjenester i Nord med et blikk på sykepleiens utvikling og bidrag. In: Tidsskrift for Nordisk Helsetjenesteforskning 9 no 1 (2013), pp. 105–123. DOI: http://dx.doi.org/10.7557/14.2568

Fause, Åshild: The fate of the mentally ill during the Second World War (1940–1945) in Troms and Finnmark, Norway. In: Nordlit 37 (2015), pp. 1–29. DOI: http://dx.doi.org/10.7557/13.3638

Fygle, Svein: Marmor og menneskeskjebner, Rønvik sykehus i det 20-århundret. Bodø 2002.

Heinrichs, I.: Sindsygepleien i dens gruntræk. Kristiania 1914.

Hvalvik, Sigrun: Bergljot Larsson og den moderne sykepleien. Oslo 2005.

Pedersen, Per B: Deinstitusjonaliseringen av det psykiske helsevernet. In: Norvoll, R. (red.): Samfunn og psykiske lidelser. Samfunnsvitenskapelige perspektiver – en introduksjon. Oslo 2002, pp. 187–204.

Kjelstadli, Knut: Fortida er ikke det den en gang var. En innføring i historiefaget. Oslo 1999.

Leikvam, Jon: Pleiepersonalets arbeidsforhold ved asylene. In : Socialistisk Medicinsk Tidsskrift Vol 2 (1935), pp. 34–39.

Lia, Gaute: Utsettelse av sinnssyke i privatpleie – En undersøkelse av familiepleien i Manger 1880–1920. Hovedfagsoppgave i historie, Universitetet i Bergen 2003.

Ludvigsen, Kari: Kunnskap og politikk i norsk sinnssykevesen1820–1920. Bergen: Rapport nr 63, Universitetet i Bergen 1998.

Martinsen, Kari: Huset, sangen, gråten og skammen. Rom og arkitektur som ivaretaker av menneskers verdighet i Trygve Wyller red): Skam. Perspektiver på skam og skamløshet i det moderne. Bergen 2001.

Mathialainen, Dahly: Idemönster i Karin Neuman-Rahn livsgärning och författerskap: en idëhistorisk-biografisk studie i psykiatrisk vård i Finland under 1900-tallets fôrsta hälft. Åbo 1997.

Neuman-Rahn, Karin: Den psykiskt sjuka människan och hennes vård. Helsingfors 1924.

Nissen, Rikke: Lærebok i sygepleie for diakoniser. Oslo 2000.

Saastad, Arve: Er god pleie av psykiatriske pasienter avhengig av profesjoner eller mennes-
ker? Utdanningsspørsmålet på Gaustad sykehus i historisk perspektiv. In: Retterstøl, Nils:
Gaustad sykehus 140 år. Oslo 1995. pp. 86–107.

Sandmo, Erling: Et uvisst sted. In: Thorvald Steen (red): Asylet. Gastad sykehus 150 år. Oslo
2005. pp. 52–74.

Sjøstrøm, Bengt: Kliniken tar over dårskapen. Om den moderna svenska psykiatrins fram-
vext. Gøteborg 1992.

Skram, Amalie: Professor Hieronimus. København 1977.

Skram, Amalie: På Sct.Jørgen. København 1977.

Skålevåg, Svein A: System i galskapen – teori og terapi i norske sinnssykeasyl, 1855–1915.
Hovedfagsoppgave i Historie, Universitetet i Bergen 1998.

Skålevåg, Svein A.: Fra normalitetens historie. Sinnssykdom 1870–1920. Bergen 2003.

Slettan, Dagfinn: Minner og kulturhistorie. Teoretiske perspektiver. Historisk Institutt, Skrift-
serie nr 4, Universitetet i Trondheim 1994.

Stave, Gunnar: Mannsmot og tenarsinn: Det Norske Diakonhjem i hundre år. Oslo 1990.

Psychiatric Nurses: An Invisible Role in the Transition between the General Hospitals and the Community[1]

Sandra Harrisson

Summary

Ontario (Canada) committed to the process of deinstitutionalization following the publication of the report, *More for the Mind* in 1963. This report recommended reducing the number of institutionalized patients in the provincial psychiatric hospitals and instigated the opening of acute care units in general hospitals for the care of patients with mental disorders. During this transitional period toward community care, several short-stay psychiatric departments opened in the general hospitals. This transition of care increased the demand for psychiatric nurses in the community. These nurses had to adapt to the new acute care setting and to prepare patients for an early return to their home. The psychiatric nurses had to redefine their role and their professional identity within the health care team as the treatment of patients underwent this transition. The nurses' observations, as recorded in the nursing notes, contributed to the treatment plans and the discharge planning of psychiatric patients.

Introduction

Years ago, the care of psychiatric patients constituted confinement inside institutions for a long period of time. Quite often, patients stayed in the asylum for a large part of their life, experimenting occasionally with short leaves with their families. The deinstitutionalization movement promoted community care as an alternative to the traditional asylum model. For the past 40 years, the province of Ontario (Canada), has attempted to transfer psychiatric care outside institutional walls with the purpose of socially reintegrating people with mental disorders into the community. During this transitional period toward community care, several short-stay psychiatric departments opened in the general hospitals to provide care for those individuals. This transition of care increased the demand for specialized health care professionals. Among these, psychiatric nurses had a central role, adapting to the new acute care setting and preparing patients for an early return to their home in the community.

My study, based on the medical records of psychiatric patients and admission records of the Psychiatric Department at the Montfort Hospital in Ot-

1   The author gratefully acknowledge the financial support of the Nursing History Research Unit (NHRU-URHN), Chaire de recherche sur la francophonie canadienne en santé, IRSC – Projet "Champ francophone de la désinstitutionnalisation en santé mentale", Réseau de recherche appliquée sur la santé des francophones en Ontario (RRASFO), MESRS – université.
    I would like to thank Marie-Claude Thifault and Jayne Elliot for the review of this paper and their support on this project, the Montfort archives managers and the research assistants for their precious collaboration.

tawa, Ontario, between 1976 and 2006, offers a new analysis of this transformation. A socio-historical perspective will be used to understand the transinstitutional trajectory of patients with chronic mental disorders in a French language minority context. The access to active[2] and inactive patient charts brings a new understanding of the history of psychiatry, dehospitalization of the mentally ill and the nurse's role in the short-term psychiatric units.

The deinstitutionalization movement compelled psychiatric nurses to redefine their role and their professional identity within the health care team as the treatment of patients underwent a paradigm shift. Nurses' expertise in chronic mental care contributed to the development of acute psychiatric care in general hospitals. The nurses' observations of patient behaviours, as recorded in the nursing notes, influenced the treatment plans and the discharge planning of patients to the community. This chapter presents a short context of the province of Ontario, the historical process of the opening of the acute care psychiatric department at Montfort Hospital, and the role of the psychiatric nurses there, including their involvement in the discharge process of the mentally ill patient.

Context

Canada is divided into ten provinces and three territories. The province of Ontario, the most populous province, is bordered by the province of Manitoba to the west and the province of Quebec to the east. Canada has two major linguistic communities, one Anglophone and the other Francophone.[3] English is the dominant language throughout the country except in the province of Quebec. Ontario has the highest percentage of Francophones in Canada, excluding Quebec. Indeed, 54% of Francophones outside Quebec are located in Ontario[4], and the majority of Franco-Ontarians live in the east of the province.

Although the city of Ottawa, in which the Montfort is located, is supposed to be bilingual, the majority of the population is English-speaking. Access to health services appeared quite difficult for Francophones until the Montfort hospital was founded in 1953 to provide health care to this population. The hospital rapidly took an important part in the Franco-Ontarian community, today is the only community hospital to provide care in the French language in eastern Ontario – significant because access to health services in one's own language is especially important for patients with a mental illness who are particularly vulnerable.[5]

---

2   In this study, the author has access to current patient's charts. Some patients in this project are still being treated in the acute-care psychiatric ward in Montfort hospital today.
3   Foucher (2010–2011), p. 54.
4   Bouchard/Desmeules (2011), pp. 5–6.
5   Harrisson/Bruyninx/MacCordick/Tessier (2015), p. 413. To learn more about the crisis concerning the attempted closure of the Montfort in 1997 and the process to reverse the

Opening of the psychiatric department in the Montfort hospital

Ontario committed to the process of deinstitutionalization following the publication of the report *More for the Mind* in 1963[6]. This report recommended reducing the number of institutionalized patients and decentralizing services that had previously been provided in the dedicated provincial psychiatric hospitals. In addition, it promoted integrating psychiatric care in general hospitals with continuing care and treatment in the community.[7-8] The report instigated the opening of acute care departments in general hospitals for the care of patients with mental disorders.

Negotiations to open such a department at the Montfort Hospital in Ottawa began in 1971. This project was approved quickly by the administrative committee and the director of the hospital under the condition of obtaining approval from the health ministry along with the necessary funds.[9] Over the next five years, M. D'Amours, the executive director at the Montfort, and Dr Blais, chief psychiatrist, developed and planned the implementation of this department of 30 psychiatric beds. I found the details of this planning in the hospital archives, such as the estimate of operational costs and equipment as well as proposed wages.

The new psychiatric department opened in 1976. Its function was "to provide a comprehensive community psychiatric service that accepts all kinds of psychiatric patients selected with no limiting criteria. The treatment setting will be short-term acute care with an early return to the community."[10] The department, using an eclectic approach in a therapeutic environment, put an emphasis on group activities,[11] which meant that all professional members of the psychiatric department had a therapeutic role and could be called on to be a therapist. Thus, different approaches and therapeutic techniques were accepted and promoted according to patient needs.

The personnel consisted of one multidisciplinary team per ten hospitalized patients. It was composed of one each of a psychiatrist, psychologist, social worker, and occupational therapist, with the rest being psychiatric nurses.[12] The goal was to establish a balanced team, although the number of

government's decision, please refer to Gratton (2003). The Hospital remained open based on the rights of Francophones to receive health services in French.

6   Tyhurst et al. (1963). This report is the precursor of psychiatric care in the community in Ontario. It followed the global trend toward deinstitutionalization arguing that patients who need short-term psychiatric care can be treated in general hospitals and then returned to the community.

7   Greenland/Griffin/Hoffman (2001), pp. 7–8.

8   This segment defines the term "dehospitalization".

9   Montfort Archives, Letter addressed to M. D'Amours from M. Teasdale, Chairman Hospital Planning Committee, June 29, 1971.

10 Montfort Archives, Document draft – compagnie architectes Agnew, Peckham & Associates LTD, May 1972.

11 Montfort Archives, Document "Sketched Program", not dated.

12 Montfort Archives, Document "procédures et règlements du département de psychiatrie", January 9th, 1975, p. 4.

nurses was larger in the short-term psychiatric department than in other disciplines. This team followed people with a mental illness in their journey through community services, that is, the day center, the external clinic and the general hospital, if they needed to be admitted.

The role of acute-care psychiatric nurses

The transition of psychiatric services between provincial psychiatric hospitals and the community has been somewhat studied. There is some research on the transformation of the role of nursing in the community,[13] but few authors have been interested in the new role of psychiatric nurses in the general hospital setting. I was determined to overcome this lack of information, but unfortunately, I was faced with an absence of data on this subject. Indeed, nurses' notes between 1976 and 1988 at Montfort Hospital were systematically destroyed in the microfiche version of inpatient records to address the storage problem of a large number of paper files. This destruction caused the loss of a great deal of historical evidence of the evolution of the nursing role during the early stage of deinstitutionalization. As Boschma has mentioned, "nurses have often left little written evidence of their practice."[14] However, the Montfort archives contained, in the section that dealt with the development of the psychiatric department, examples of the forms used for nursing notes and care plans. Some of the care plans demonstrated the revisions necessary as the patient's condition and needs constantly evolved. These documents illustrated individual nursing care and were a reminder of nursing interventions, lab work and other tests scheduled for each patient. Care plans were also used as a tool for communication between nursing personnel.[15] Little else remains from that period, however, that represents nursing work. During the data collection, the care plan was not included in the database because of their random frequency. However, the nurses' notes were left on the patients' files after 1988 and thus I was able to use those from that date until 2006 in this study to help to understand the role of psychiatric nurses in the acute care unit.

Charles Hanly, in his 1970 report *Mental Health in Ontario*,[16] explained the current state of mental health care and services in the province and made some recommendations to the Ministry of Health. At the beginning of his report, he introduced two different views of mental health care. The first view adopted the ideal that everything possible must be done to assure that each individual has the support necessary to obtain a healthy mental state. The second view is quite the opposite, guaranteeing care only to the severely ill who could endanger themselves or others in contact with them. For the re-

---

13   For more information on this subject, please refer to Boschma (2012); Boschma/Groening/Boyd (2008); Boschma/Mychajilunow (2005); Church (1986).
14   Boschma (2012), p. 106.
15   Blackwood Kozier / Witter DuGas (1967), p. 146.
16   Hanly (1970).

mainder of people with a mental illness, their family and community should provide care and accommodation. It was thought that only a small number of people would require specialized mental health care. Hanly recommended in his report the establishment of a realistic goal between the utopian maximum and the traditional minimum.

During this period, the health network in Ontario was facing a shortage of psychiatrists and other mental health professionals.[17] Hanly recognized that nursing in general was undergoing a transformation as a result of several factors such as a strong pressure toward specialization, a diminished need for general nursing and a shortage of nurses. Nevertheless, he believed that

> two basic features of traditional nursing still prevail and are likely to prevail in the future: (1) in Ontario, nursing is essentially a woman's profession and; (2) the nurse is the one person who is involved in all aspects of the patient's care and well-being on an hourly and daily basis during hospitalization.[18]

For him the function of the nurse in psychiatric settings was identical with that of nurses on a non-psychiatric ward:

> The (1) supervision and/or provision of the general care of the patient; (2) dispensing of drugs being used in the treatment; (3) performance of routine medical checks when they are required; (4) ongoing observation of the progress of the patient and his treatment and (5) cooperation with other professional staff involved in the diagnosis and the treatment of the patient in the formation of a workable treatment program.[19]

Hanly added that the psychiatric nurse might engage in a supportive and therapeutic relationship with the patient and develop personalized care on an individual basis.[20] But his description of psychiatric nurses does not reflect the entire scope of the responsibilities and expertise of those nurses.

The work of Hildegard Peplau, founder of modern psychiatric nursing, is helpful to understand the role of psychiatric nurses. In her first book, *Interpersonal Relations in Nursing: A Conceptual Frame of Reference for Psychodynamic Nursing,*[21] she conceptualized the process of the nurse-patient interaction, advancing the idea that these interpersonal phenomena have a qualitative impact on patient outcome.[22] She imagined that this distinct therapeutic role for nursing, oriented toward developing an interpersonal relationship, would help to understand the psychosocial behavioural problems of the patient rather than focusing on the mental illness diagnosis. According to Peplau, "interpersonal relations concepts provide a framework for understanding many of the dilem-

---

17 Hanly (1970), p. 3.
18 Hanly (1970), p. 141.
19 Hanly (1970), p. 142.
20 Hanly (1970), p. 143.
21 Peplau (1952). The first edition of her book was published in 1952 and reissued in 1991. The later editions remained similar of the original work except the preface written by the author. In this note, she recognized that "for the past decades, interpersonal theory has been greatly expanded by nursing research and social sciences" and "this book remains a useful foundation" for nurses (1991, p. vi).
22 Peplau (1952); Callaway (2002).

mas that patients experience [and these lie] within the domain of professional nursing practice."[23] Her theory assists nurses to make sense of patients' experience and behaviour related to their health and illness, including mental illness.[24] The development of her theoretical work coincided with the transition of care for mentally ill patients to the community setting and to short-term units in general hospitals. Today, Peplau's theory is taught in nursing programs all over the world as part of general knowledge for nurses, and not only as part of the psychiatric curriculum.[25] In fact, "the nurse-patient relationship has become the center of nursing practice".[26]

In the mid-20th century, the practice of psychiatric nursing faced major changes. Some nurses and psychiatrists resisted the increased independence of psychiatric nursing practice but others joined in developing this new nursing role. Several articles were written about this new trend of developing psychiatric nursing in the psychiatric hospital and the community[27] but few authors were interested in the short-term psychiatric units in general hospitals. In her book, *The Psychiatric Nurse in the General Hospital*,[28] written in 1959, Mary Tudbury introduced the practice of psychiatric nursing in the short-term unit setting in the United States. Her book was described as a practical guide for clinical nurses who wanted to practice in psychiatry. Strongly influenced by Hildegard Peplau, Tudbury promoted the development of the interpersonal nurse-client relationship and nurses' active role in the establishment of a therapeutic environment in the acute care unit. For Tudbury, a psychiatric nurse

> is interested in the patient as a person and is desirous of helping him by total nursing care; that is, she is cognizant of the fact that knowledge of and an ability to apply technical skills alone does not constitute good nursing care. The nurse recognizes the need for the human side of nursing, those things over and above the mechanical.[29]

She addressed the problem of the rapid turnover of patients in the general hospital and, consequently, the shorter periods of time available to establish a therapeutic relationship compared to the typical mental hospital. Moreover, she encouraged nurses to take an active role in the multidisciplinary team and to be more than the executioner of the doctor's orders.

Many psychiatrists requested nurses with specific psychiatric experience to work on the acute psychiatric wards of general hospitals. They believed that general registered nurses lacked psychiatric knowledge. In the majority of Canadian nursing schools in the 1970s theoretical psychiatric courses had

---

23 Peplau (1997), p. 162.
24 Peplau (1997), p. 162.
25 Senn (2013), pp. 31–35, illustrated Peplau's theory in other nursing specialities such as emergency room or rural nursing.
26 D'Antonio/Beeber/Sills/Naegle (2014), p. 312.
27 To read about the evolution of the psychiatric nurse's role in the 1950's, refer to Bennett/ Eaton (1951); Black (1952); Kandler/Behymer/Kegeles/Boyd (1952); Kremsdorf (1951); Mereness (1951).
28 Tudbury (1959).
29 Tudbury (1959), p. 58.

been decreased to under 45 hours.[30] One cause of this change was connected to the transition of hospital nursing schools to colleges or universities. However, it is important to note that in the 1970s, the term "psychiatric nurse" was commonly used in three different ways.[31] The first category referred to a graduate registered nurse working with mentally ill patients in a hospital setting, although there was no school in Ontario where a general nurse could receive advanced training in a psychiatric specialty. The second category described graduates from psychiatric training programs offered in the Canadian western provinces, or in Jamaica or Great Britain. The last category was nurses who graduated from schools that were not recognized by Ontario. Of the three categories, the preferred one was registered nurses with psychiatric experience because their general medical knowledge was useful in treating the diverse health problems of mentally ill patients, whether they were inside provincial psychiatric hospitals, general hospitals or out in the community. However, some psychiatrists believed it took between six months to a year to train a registered nurse in psychiatric nursing.[32]

When reading the documents on the development of the operational plan of the Montfort psychiatric department, it was clear that there were some problems recruiting qualified Francophone physicians. Indeed, there are few job opportunities listed in the 1975 journals and newspapers.[33] The Montfort Hospital tried to recruit French speaking psychiatrists from other Francophone or bilingual provinces such as Quebec and New Brunswick. Recruiting Francophone psychiatric nurses also seemed to be a problem. In a letter addressed to M. Teasdale, Chairman of the Hospital Planning Committee, M. D'Amours asked if it would be possible to recruit some nurses affiliated with the Montfort School of Nursing as early as 1971.[34]

It is difficult to determine where the French-speaking psychiatric nurses came from since specific documents on their recruitment are closed. With the coming of deinstitutionalization, it is very likely that a number of nurses from provincial psychiatric hospitals transferred to the acute care units in general hospitals, and some of these undoubtedly ended up at the Montfort. The closest institution to the Montfort for chronic mentally ill patients was the psychi-

---

30 Hanly (1970); Rainville/Bourdon (1986).
31 Hanly (1970), pp. 141–142.
32 Hanly (1970), p. 147.
33 Montfort Archives, advertisements in an unknown newspaper for French psychiatrists dated 10-11-1975 and December 1975. Furthermore, we found a note of service (20-01-1975) written by Dr Blais stating that advertisement for French psychiatrists has been posted in Newspapers such as *Le Devoir*, *Le Jour* and *La Presse* and would be posted in medical journals such as *Union Médicale* and *Revue de l'Association des Psychiatres du Canada*.
34 Montfort Archives, Letter addressed to M. D. N. Teasdale, Chairman Hospital Planning Committee from M. D'Amours dated July 6th, 1971. The psychiatric unit plan included the architectural and financial plan, the staffing and the materials needed. Even if the unit did not open until 1976, the Hospital Planning Committee was anticipating some difficulty in recruiting French mental health professionals as early as 1971. The proximity of the Montfort School of Nursing was an important asset for the administrators from which to recruit French registered nurses to work on the new psychiatric unit.

atric hospital in Brockville, a community about 100 km away, which remains in operation today. Mental health services were primarily provided in English in this institution even if over 400 residents were Francophone by the end of 1960s.[35]

Nevertheless, these nurses, in redefining their roles in these new psychiatric acute care settings, constituted themselves from the experience they had developed over the years with chronic mentally ill patients in long-term care facilities. According to Boschma,

> psychiatric nurses, trained in the mental hospital, carried their experience with them to the new places they constructed [...] In the construction of these new services, nurses were able to carve out a new professional identity that expanded their independence, therapeutic role, and capacity for leadership.[36]

For example, nurses in the psychiatric hospitals had started to prepare their patients for discharge before the 1960s, developing different types of therapies such as group and individual interventions and milieu therapy[37] to create a healing environment. They certainly took this experience and knowledge with them in creating their new role in the short-term psychiatric departments in general hospitals.

Psychiatric nurses: Participation in the patient discharge planning

After 1988, the nurse's notes of the short-term psychiatric department at the Montfort help us understand the role of psychiatric nurses in discharge planning. By that time, the forms "Nursing Evaluation" and the nurses' notes themselves are present in patients' paper charts. Those notes reflect the fundamental needs of the psychiatric patients, their mental status, their relationship with the outside world and their reactions to temporary discharges. The records reveal, in some cases, examples of developing relationships between patients and nurses during therapeutic interviews. However, when reading those notes, the nurses appear most of the time distant, even invisible, in the caring process of these patients. Yet, they have a central role in the care of the mentally ill on the psychiatric unit and are involved in the discharge planning for outside the hospital walls. The overall impression is that nurses are relegated to a supporting role for other health professionals.

---

35 Asylum Projects (2014).
36 Boschma (2012), p. 116, 128.
37 Several authors wrote about milieu therapy in the 1960s and 1970s, see Rioc/Stanton (1953); Artiss (1962); Eldred/Vanderpol (1968); Almond (1974) (this list is not exhaustive). As per LeCuyer (1992), milieu therapy is an interdisciplinary theoretical and clinical approach to inpatient psychiatric treatment in which the total environment has a therapeutic potential. It was developed in long-term facilities. The psychiatric nurses had to adapt this therapy in the acute psychiatric unit in general hospitals. The implementation of the short stays modified the goals of the milieu therapy. The new goals include crisis intervention, symptom stabilization, restoration of previous functioning, and longer length of community tenure before rehospitalization.

Nurses contribute to the establishment of the diagnosis, the plan of care and the treatment by writing their observations in the patient's chart. They are responsible for the patient's medical record, which is a concise written account of all the information concerning the patient, containing the patient's history, examinations, tests, diagnosis, prognosis, therapy and response to treatments. It serves as a means of communication among all health professionals involved with the patient.[38] The purpose of the chart has not changed in many years. Even in 1939,[39] nursing books mentioned its importance. Its multiple purposes include: 1) to help the doctor to establish a diagnosis and treatment and to follow the evolution of the disease; 2) to compile the documents necessary for statistics; 3) to stimulate scientific research; 4) to consult in certain legal claims; 5) to save unnecessary costs of examinations and tests when the patient has been previously hospitalized.[40]

Between 1988 and 2006, the patient's record at the Montfort contained similar documents and retained the same structure over the period under study. The first section contained the administrative papers followed by the discharge summary and the admission requests filled by the doctor, which, in our case, were mostly for psychiatrists and sometimes internal medicine physicians. The next section contained all the information relating to the emergency room: the emergency report, the triage and the emergency nursing. If the patient had been transferred from another hospital, the transfer request and all documents related to the patient's stay are inserted in that same section. The rest of the chart contained information about the patient's hospitalization, such as the medical history, physical examination, doctor's orders, progress notes completed by doctors and others health professionals such as social workers, psychologists and occupational therapists, consultations, laboratory reports, vital signs chart, medication sheets, the nursing evaluation form completed during the first hours of admission to the psychiatric department, nursing notes and the care plan. This represents only one hospitalization. In fact, this process of chart construction is repeated with each admission. The patient's chart may appear simply an accumulation of information but it actually is a useful tools for communication among different health professionals in the psychiatric care of the hospitalized patient.

The nursing notes make up an important part of the constitution of the patient's chart. Blackwood Kozier and Witter DuGas, in their 1967 book *Fundamentals of Patient Care: A Comprehensive Approach to Nursing,* provided directives on how to write good quality nursing notes, which are helpful in analyzing the nursing notes at the Montfort. In general, nurses' notes are used to convey five categories of information:

---

38 The construction of medical record and its purpose remain mainly unchanged. Harmer/ Henderson (1939); Soeurs de la Charité / Soeurs Grises de Montréal (1947); Blachwood Kozier / Witter DuGas (1967).

39 Harmer/Henderson (1939).

40 Sœurs de la Charité / Sœurs Grises de Montréal (1947).

1) therapeutic measures carried out by various members of the health team; 2) measures ordered by the physician and carried out by nursing personnel; 3) nursing measures which are not ordered by the physician but which the nurse carries out to meet the specific needs of a patient; 4) behavior of the patient which is considered to be pertinent to his general health; 5) specific responses of the patient to therapy and care.[41]

The nurses also record visits from the doctor or other health professionals, whether or not physician's orders have been carried out, and if not, the reason why. Because this type of charting records the care and therapies carried out by all members of the health team, including the doctor and the nurses, it serves as a communication tool for the entire medical staff.

One of the psychiatric nurse's responsibilities is to record the behaviour of the patient considered pertinent to his general health, which includes the physiological reaction to illness or treatment but also his or her emotional tone, verbal communication and physical action. According to Harmer and Henderson, "[the nurse] must observe and record and often interpret physical and mental manifestations of health and disease, and she must be critical of and alter conditions in the environment that affect the patient's well-being."[42] These are the only authors advocating for nurses to interpret patients' behaviours. Other nursing practice textbooks underline the importance of uninterpreted reporting of nurses' observations.[43] In fact, opinions and interpretations of patient's behaviour are usually omitted.[44]

Nonetheless, nurses decide what needs to be reported in nursing notes, and their decisions have a major impact on the establishment of diagnosis, treatment and discharge planning. The psychiatrist depends on this information to create an individual treatment plan. Hanly recognized that the nurse has the most contact with the patient and therefore has the major responsibility for keeping the patient's progress under informed observation to provide and supervise his general care.[45] Even if the nursing notes do not reflect the magnitude of the nurses' work, when reading them we can see the total picture of patient progress toward a partial or sometimes a total recovery, along with some nurses' interventions.

Observation is an essential part of the nurse's responsibilities. The nurse must recognize the signs and symptoms of physical and mental health and find out the factors influencing normal or abnormal development of an individual, the specific symptoms of each disease, the patient's reactions to prescribed and non-prescribed medications and treatments, and the amelioration or deterioration of his health.[46] Symptoms are divided into two categories: subjective and objective. The subjective symptoms are only perceptible by the

---

41   Sœurs de la Charité / Sœurs Grises de Montréal (1947), p. 145.
42   Harmer/Henderson (1939), p. 6.
43   Even today, nursing students are directed to write their observations without interpretation or personal opinion. They are to write only the facts, and the objective and subjective signs and symptoms.
44   Blackwood Kozier / Witter DuGas (1967), p. 146.
45   Hanly (1970).
46   Sœurs de la Charité / Sœurs Grises de Montréal (1947), p. 267.

patient and are not externally visible. When the nurse reports these symptoms on the chart, she quotes the patient's description without interpretation
of the data. The objective symptoms can be observed by others. The nurse
will write, in her notes, the observations of the patient's mental or physical
behaviours that she thinks might affect the diagnosis, the treatment, the nursing care or the discharge planning.[47]

One patient's psychiatric journey at the Montfort Hospital

To illustrate these points, I will refer to one patient, selected because the nursing notes are complete and reflect the content of the majority of patient records. Diagnosed with schizophrenia, Irene[48] was admitted 25 times to the
psychiatric department between 1976 and 1999 for a total of 1337 days of
hospitalization. Her stays varied between 23 to 97 days. She was French-Ca-
nadian, married with two sons, and lived close to Ottawa city limits. Her husband was very supportive and involved in her care and well-being, present
throughout his wife's psychiatric journey at the hospital.

Analysis of the nurse's notes allows for understanding the significance of
the observations written in the patient's chart as decision-making progressed
on the multidisciplinary treatment plan and the psychiatrist's decision to ap-
prove a definite discharge. This observation started upon the patient's arrival
on the acute ward. The admission entry describes the reason for the patient's
arrival on the department, his or her emotional state and whether or not the
person is accompanied by family or a friend or came alone.

Irene's admission in 1994 was her 18th visit to the short-term unit. She was
55 years old at that time and well known to the staff. The first entry notes are
as follows:

> 14-06-1994 (22h00) – Pt admitted to floor ambulatory accompanied by son. [Vital signs
> (VS)] taken. Personal effects searched. Personal history taken with help from son – pt
> unable to answer most questions – unable to comprehend. Pt cooperative during inter-
> view with son present. Paranoid ideas present – not allowing certain staff members to
> approach her. Often asking for food – saying she is very hungry. Pt repetitive in her de-
> mands but calm. (23h00) Walking in hallway with beverage in her hands.[49]

During the initial contact with the patient, the nurse is assessing the patient's
different needs. For example, the nurse takes vital signs and searches personal
effects to ensure that all security measures are taken before accompanying the
patient to her room. This search is routine, and is done systematically every
time the patient leaves the unit for any period of time. The fact that the patient
is accompanied by her son gives a first impression of family involvement. In
this case, the son's positive influence helps the admitting nurse complete the

---

47   Harmer/Henderson (1939), p. 273.
48   A fictive name that I personally gave to this patient.
49   Reference no. pt2181.id9218.nn.pdf. Please note that Pt refers to the word patient and
     VS to vital signs.

"Nursing Evaluation" questionnaire. The patient is more cooperative and calm with her son by her side. However, Irene seems distressed upon admission, with the nurse noting some concentration difficulties, paranoid ideation and mistrust of some the staff. The initial observation of mental status is important to assist the entire psychiatric team meet Irene's physical, sociological and psychological needs during her hospital stay.[50] The team can already anticipate the patient will return home with her family when ready for discharge.

During the course of Irene's hospitalization, the nurses wrote about her mood, her feelings or what they deemed her appropriate or inappropriate behaviours. During her hospitalization in 1994, Irene was quite hostile and suspicious of the staff. On her fourth day, the nurse wrote:

> 17-06-1994 (15h30–23h30) Pt walking in hallway on arrival with towel on top of her head – hostile toward nurse – saying that she doesn't want me near her. Suspicious about her 17h00 meds – said that they were not the right meds + wanted to take all of her meds for the day. Pt dressed in blue gown + housecoat, did not complain of the heat. Pt often at front desk during evening requesting meds – remained suspicious + hostile. Did not eat supper – said she was on a diet – drank well throughout evening.

Because Irene has a towel on her head and is quite overdressed for the temperature on the unit, the nurse believed she demonstrated inadequate behaviour. During the day, Irene had been suffering from the heat because of the heat wave, and the staff was quite worried about her risk of dehydration. But her behaviour changed during the evening and she doesn't dress appropriately now. Furthermore, she is still hostile and suspicious toward the personnel but at the same time it seemed that she needed to feel safe by spending some time at the nursing front desk.

One month later, the day nurse reported:

> 14-07-1994 (07h30–15h30) Up at 10h35, goes immediately to her activity (crafts). Ate well at lunch. At pm, agrees to get dressed and goes outside with her nursing assistant. Asked to return a second time. When back, called her husband to ask him to come visit her. No suspicious or hostile mood noted. More independent.[51]

This is the first report of Irene's improvement, but although she participated in different activities and seemed less isolated, the next reports are still focused on her inappropriate behaviours and her abnormal mental status. Not until a week later did the nurses note more constant amelioration of her mental status. Her mood is more stable and she begins to socialize with other patients. She is more autonomous in her carrying out her personal hygiene and she is cooperative about her care. She starts talking about her family and expresses some sad feelings.

> 22-07-1994 (15h30–23h30) Dressed. Mood stable. Socialized with us. Went for a walk outside alone. Ate her supper. Cleaned her clothes on her own initiative. Husband visited. Went to walk outside with him. Happy. Calm. Asked about possible weekend pass.[52]

---

50 Blackwood Kozier / Witter DuGas (1967), p. 37.
51 The nursing notes are written in French or English at the nurse convenience because Montfort Hospital has a bilingual status. This note is a free translation by the author.
52 Free translation.

The nurses must report some steady improvement of Irene's mental status before she can be considered eligible for a pass to go home. A week later, she obtained permission to spend a few hours at home. Irene and her husband planned the short leave with the nursing staff, and she left in the morning to return to her home environment for few hours.

> 31-07-1994 (07h30–15h30) Got up at 08h00. In a good mood. Very adequate and comfortable. Leaves for the day with her husband at 10h00. […] Will return at 22h00. Back at 19h45 with her husband. Smiling, relaxed. States had a good day at home.[53]

Some patients are anxious about the first short stay at home, often understanding that being away from the house for a few days and even weeks may put some stress on their families. By the time patients are eligible for a pass, their mental status is normally improving. Still, the result of the time away from the unit will have an impact on the length of their hospitalization. If the results were positive, the patient could obtain several weekend passes or even her discharge, otherwise, the hospital stay may be prolonged.

At Irene's return, the nurse evaluated the effect of this short stay in her home environment, noting the significant improvement in her mood and behaviour. The nurse wrote that she was in a good mood, socialized with other patients, had a good level of energy, was calm and cooperative and took care of her appearance. Irene also started to talk about the impact of her illness on her family. The day after her short leave, she was already planning her next weekend at home.

During hospitalization, psychiatric nurses observe the interaction between the patient and family members and record their visits as part of the process of discharge planning. Close family involvement, or the lack of it, gives a clear indication of the possibility of the patient's return home or whether placement in a group home or a residence would be better. In Irene's case, the nursing notes reflect the frequent visits of by her husband. For example:

> 13-07-1994 19h00 Husband in visiting – out to walk on hospital grounds with him.

Activities carried out during family visits, as well as the patient's positive or negative reactions to the visit, can also be added. Occasionally, the nursing notes reveal a partnership between nursing staff and the family member in some therapeutic interventions.

> 03-07-1994 (07h30–15h30) Remains motionless in her bed for long periods of time […] Keeping complete silence in my presence. 13h30. Husband's visit on the unit. Suggestion made to her husband to attempt to mobilize her and do some activities during his visit.[54]

Following the nurse's intervention, Irene's husband took her on frequent walks on the hospital grounds and to a nearby shopping mall, and out for occasional dinners at a restaurant.

> 19-07-1994 18h30 Husband in visiting – said he was taking [his wife] out for supper – advised that she had already eaten. Return at 20h00. In good spirits – smiling.

---

53   Free translation.
54   Free translation.

The collaborative work between nursing staff and Irene's husband prepares Irene and her family for leaves and eventually permanent discharge. Irene obtained a total of three weekend passes before she was able to return home.

The psychiatrist seemed to be influenced by the nurses' observation written in the patient's chart. In fact, the medical exit notes reflect the progress noted by the nurses during Irene's hospitalization. The psychiatrist summarizes, in just a few words, what the nurses describe on a daily basis. After noticing a significant improvement in the patient's health and confirming this observation with those made by the nurses, the psychiatrist authorizes the patient's final release on August 11th.

> 11-08-1994 [...] The evolution of the patient in the department has been very slow. The patient gradually displayed a better contact with reality, her behaviours became more appropriate. Her childish behaviour disappeared. Her mental state has stabilized and she was discharge from the hospital, improved. She will be followed in the outpatient clinic.[55]

Irene had stayed 58 days in the short-term psychiatric unit during this hospitalization, reflecting the journey of the majority of patients admitted to the same unit.

The nursing notes and their observations directly influenced the care and the discharge planning of those individuals and their return to the community.

Conclusion

The destruction of nurse's notes contributes to the loss of collective memory in our understanding of the transition process of mental health care and services to the community. These notes, written between 1976 and 1987, could have revealed the organization and evolution of nursing care on the short-stay psychiatric department. However, nurses' notes do not necessarily do justice to the nurse's place within the multidisciplinary or interdisciplinary team, rarely indicating the multiple nursing interventions carried out by nurses for their patients. Yet, when I analyzed this set of notes, I realized that nurses took their place among the other mental health professionals by establishing a therapeutic environment in the acute care setting through interpersonal interactions with patients. Indeed, nurses decided which observations and critical information were relevant and must be recorded in the patient's chart, which, in turn, had a major influence on the decision process and the development of the treatment plan devised by the other mental health professionals and the psychiatrist.

I believe that this part of nursing history deserves further consideration to fill the gap in the historiography of nursing and the development of community psychiatric services. Actually, it would be quite interesting to complete this part of nursing history and finally make more visible these psychiatric care pioneers.

---

55   Free translation of the psychiatrist discharge note.

Bibliography

Archival sources

Montfort Archives

Letter addressed to M. D'Amours from M. Teasdale, Chairman Hospital Planning Committee, June 29, 1971.

Letter addressed to M.D.N. Teasdale, Chairman Hospital Planning Committee from M. D'Amours dated July 6th, 1971.

Document draft – compagnie architectes Agnew, Peckham & Associates LTD, May 1972.

Document "Sketched Program", not dated.

Document "procédures et règlements du département de psychiatrie", January 9th, 1975.

Montfort medical records, patient's chart reference #2181.id9218.

Secondary research literature

Almond, Richard: The Healing Community: Dynamics of the Therapeutic Milieu. New York 1974.

Artiss, Kenneth L.: Milieu Therapy in Schizophrenia. New York 1962.

Asylum Project. Brockville Asylum for the insane 2014 http://www.asylumprojects.org/index.php?title=Brockville_Asylum_for_the_insane

Bennett, A. E.; Eaton, June T.: The Role of the Psychiatric Nurse in the Newer Therapies. In: American Journal of Psychiatry 108 (1951), pp. 167–170.

Black, Kathleen: Appraising the Psychiatric Patient's Nursing Needs. In: American Journal of Nursing 52(6) (1952), pp. 718–721.

Blackwood Kozier, Barbara; Witter DuGas, Beverly: Fundamentals of Patient Care, a Comprehensive Approach to Nursing. Philadelphia; London 1967.

Boschma, Geertje: Community Mental Health Nursing in Alberta, Canada: An Oral History. In: Nursing History Review 20 (2012), pp. 103–135.

Boschma, Geertje; Groening, Marlee; Boyd Mary Ann: Psychiatric and Mental Health Nursing from Past to Present. In: Austin, Wendy; Boyd, Mary Ann (ed.): Psychiatric Nursing for Canadian Practice. Lippincott 2008, pp. 3–17.

Boshma, Geertje; Yonge, O.; Mychajilunow, L.: Gender and Professional Identity in Psychiatric Nursing Practice in Alberta, Canada, 1930–1975. In: Nursing Inquiry 12(4) (2005), pp. 243–255.

Bouchard, Louise; Desmeules, Martin: Minorités de langue officielle du Canada: Égales devant la santé? Presses de l'Université du Québec 2011.

Callaway, Barbara J.: Hildegard Peplau, Psychiatric Nurse of the Century. New York 2002.

Church, Olga Maranjian: From Custody to Community in Psychiatric Nursing. In: Nursing Research 36 (1986), 1, pp. 48–55.

D'Antonio, Patricia; Beeber, Linda; Sills, Grayce; Naegle, Madeline: The Future in the Past: Hildegard Peplau and Interpersonal Relations in Nursing. In: Nursing Inquiry 21 (2014), 4, pp. 311–317.

Eldred, Stanley H.; Vanderpol, Maurice: Psychotherapy in the Designed Therapeutic Milieu. Boston 1968.

Foucher, Pierre: Francophone minoritaire en droit canadien: une question de choix? In: Revue du Nouvel-Ontario, 35–36 (2010–2011), pp. 47–67.

Gratton, Michel: Montfort. La lutte d'un people. Centre Franco-Ontarien des Ressources pédagogiques 2003.

Greenland, Cyril; Griffin, Jack D.; Hoffman, Brian F.: Psychiatry in Canada from 1952 to 2001. In: Rae-Grant, Quentin (ed.): Psychiatry in Canada: 50 Years. Canadian Psychiatric Association 2001, pp. 1–16.

Hanly, Charles: Mental Health in Ontario. A Study for the Committee on the Healing Arts. Ontario 1970.

Harrisson, Sandra; Bruyninx, Gladys; MacCordock, Nicolas M. H.; Tessier, François: Note de recherche: Incursion dans les archives de l'Hôpital Montfort: Partir à la quête du processus de "déhospitalisation" des patients hospitalisés sur les unités psychiatriques de courte durée. In: Canadian Bulletin of Medicine History 32 (2015), 2, pp. 411–421.

Kandler, Harriet; Behymer, Alice F.; Kegeles, Stephen; Boyd, Richard W.: A Study of Nurse-Patient Interaction in a Mental Hospital. In: American Journal of Nursing 52 (1952), 9, pp. 1100–1103.

Kremsdorf, Diris: Redefining the Role of the Psychiatric Nurse. In: Nursing World 125 (1951), pp. 109–111.

LeCuyer, Elizabeth A.: Milieu Therapy for Short Stay Units. A Transformed Practice Theory. In: Archives of Psychiatric Nursing 6 (1992), 2, pp. 108–116.

Mereness, Dorothy: Preparation of the Nurse for the Psychiatric Team. In: American Journal of Nursing 51 (1951), 5, pp. 320–322.

Peplau, Hildegard: Interpersonal Relations in Nursing. A Conceptual Frame of Reference for Psychodynamic Nursing. New York 1991.

Peplau, Hildegard: Peplau's Theory of Interpersonal Relations. In: Nursing Science Quarterly 10 (1997), 4, pp. 162–167.

Rioch, David; Stanton, Alfred: Milieu Therapy. In: Psychiatry 16 (1953), 1, pp. 65–72.

Rainville, Thérèse; Bourdon, Marie-Andrée: La formation des infirmières, clé du changement? In: Santé Mentale au Québec 11 (1986), 2, pp. 59–64.

Senn, Joanne F.: Peplau's Theory of Interpersonal Relations: Application in Emergency and Rural Nursing. In: Nursing Science Quarterly 26 (2013), 1, pp. 31–35.

Smith, Mary; Khanlou, Nazilla: An Analysis of Canadian Psychiatric Mental Health Nursing through the Junctures of History, Gender, Nursing Education, and Quality of Work Life in Ontario, Manitoba, Alberta, and Saskatchewan. ISRN Nursing 2013, pp. 1–13. http://dx.doi.org/10.1155/2013/184024

Soeurs de la Charité et Soeurs Grises de Montréal: Le soin des malades, principes et techniques. Institut Marguerite d'Youville. École supérieure d'Infirmières affiliée à l'Université de Montréal 1947.

Tipliski, Veryl Margaret: Parting in the Crossroads: the Emergence of Education for Psychiatric Nursing in Three Canadian Provinces, 1909–1955. In: Canadian Bulletin of Medicine History, 21(2) (2004), pp. 253–279.

Tudbury, Mary: The Psychiatric Nurse in the General Hospital. Springfield 1959.

Tyhurst, J. S.; Chalke, F. C. R.; Lawson, F. S.; McNeel, B. H.; Roberts, C. A.; Taylor, G. C.; Weil, R. J.; Griffin, J. D.: More for the Mind. The Canadian Mental Health Association 1963.

New Contexts of Care: Work Relationships among Nurses, Patients and Volunteers in Community-Based Psychiatry in Western Canada, 1970–1990[1]

Geertje Boschma

Summary

Mental health policy shifted from a focus on large mental hospitals towards community-based services in most western countries after the 1950s. How this complex social change affected psychiatric nurses' work is not well understood. We also know little about the way patients and volunteers engaged with the construction of new community mental health services. This paper explores how community services were established using the lens of nurses', patients' and community volunteers' experiences in British Columbia, Canada, as one case example. Hence, the main question is not only how psychiatric nurses transformed their work as community care arose but also how it intersected with new patient activism and emerging peer support work. These changes occurred in the midst of public controversy over institutional psychiatry, a rising patient rights movement and a fierce anti-psychiatric critique of medical authority from the 1970s onwards, interrupting traditional nurse and patient identities .

Introduction

In this chapter I examine the shift from institutional to community mental health care in the Canadian province of British Columbia (BC) in the 1970s and 1980s, by focusing on one particular example of the establishment of a new facility for community living of discharged patients from BC's public mental hospital Riverview in the 1980s, called *Pioneer House*.[2] This facility – initially for 20, later for 30 discharged patients – was established by the Riverview Hospital Volunteer Association (RHVA), newly founded in 1980. In reality the RVHA was an extension of the existing Volunteer Department of Riverview Hospital (RH) that had existed on the hospital grounds since 1955. The radical difference, however, was that in the RVHA former patients had an essential role. The RHVA was purposely formed to create new forms of com-

1 Acknowledgement: This paper is in part drawn from G. Boschma, Community mental health post-1950: Reconsidering nurses' and consumers' identity, Routledge Handbook on the Global History of Nursing, eds. P. Antonio, J. Fairman, & J. Whelan, published by Taylor & Francis, UK Office (2013, p. 237–58) and is re-used with permission (mpkbookspermissions@tandf.co.uk).
2 This paper draws from two studies, one on the shift to community mental health in BC of which I was Principal Investigator (PI) (Funded by the Vancouver Foundation) and a multisite project on the history of deinstitutionalization in Canada (funded by Canadian Institutes of Health Research), of which I was co-investigator with PIs Megan Davies and Erika Dyck.

munity living for discharged patients *in* the community.[3] The RHVA had patient representation on its board in the person of Dave Beamish, a former
patient of Riverview Hospital, who also was a leader within the Mental Patient
Association in nearby Vancouver, BC, founded about 10 years prior.[4] Interestingly, other board members of the RVHA were members of the existing RH
Volunteer Department and psychiatric nurses. In 1980, these volunteers and
psychiatric nurses joined forces with an activist new group of more radical
"volunteers" – former patients who had taken an activist stand in Vancouver's
mental health politics. Organized as the Mental Patient Association of Vancouver (MPA) in 1971, they had successfully established a presence at RH, as
I will discuss later in the paper.[5] In 1980, these groups organized themselves
on the mental hospital grounds into the RHVA. Setting up Pioneer House in
New Westminster, BC, a city located in the vicinity of RH, was its first project.

The main goal in foregrounding this case as an example of new community services is to show, first, how a radicalized patient movement had a form-
ing influence on new forms of community care, and second, how, within this
transformation both nurses and patients renegotiated their roles and identities. The collaboration between these three groups in founding Pioneer House
seems a unique experiment in part because it was a patient and nurses-driven
facility founded on principles of rehabilitation and increased patient-control.
The group drew from a prominent example set by the radical MPA, Canada's
first patient-led organization, which was prominent in Vancouver. As an extension of their political activism, the MPA also had established a presence on
the mental hospital grounds.[6]

Scrutinizing in more detail the unusual alliance of the RHVA provides
important insights in community mental health history from a nursing and
patient point of view. The formation of the RHVA and the Pioneer House
project were part of a larger transformation of services, once confined to a
large mental hospital, into a new matrix of community services in the 1970s.
In the institution, patients and nurses might have been the least powerful
groups, but they certainly dominated by their numbers alone. In the early
1950s the patient population of RH peaked at about 4,600 patients while its
hospital-based training school took in hundreds of student psychiatric nurses
every year.[7] By zooming in on nurses' role in this transformation and the influence of the ground breaking work of patients, and on the role of a third allied,
often overlooked group of volunteer-citizens, we may attain a more nuanced
understanding of the shift to community services in the 1970s and 1980s. The
case example shows how "caring work" obtained new dimensions and re-

---

3   Riverview Hospital Volunteer Association (RHVA) (1980), Interview with Colleen Dewar
     by M. Gorrie and author, New Westminster, February 2009.
4   Interview with Dave Beamish by author, Vancouver, August 2011.
5   For a history of the MPA, see note 6.
6   MPA Founders Collective (2013).
7   Annual Report (AR), [BC] Mental Health Services Branch (MHSB) 1951, pp. 90–91.
     Hereafter cited as AR MHSB. For a discussion of the School of Psychiatric Nursing at
     RH see the section on psychiatric nurses later in the chapter.

shaped the meaning of both nursing and patient work. Pioneer House was designed to provide enduring support, work and a place to live *in* the community, not acute or short-term treatment. Enduring support and paid work continues to be the most challenging aspects of community mental health care, which makes the example significant. In the Pioneer House project, nurses and patients collaborated in transforming their work and service into new models of community care, but in so doing, they also drew on, and in a sense, renewed existing institutional structures. The somewhat unique endeavor of Pioneer House illustrates that point.

Historiography

The "community" as a domain of service beyond the institutional context has only to a limited degree been analyzed from the perspective of psychiatric nurses. Much of the existing historiography on psychiatric nursing in Canada has focused on patterns of professionalization and examined the evolution of hospital-based training of psychiatric nurses, whereas this research focuses on the way nurses transformed their work both within mental hospitals and in the changing "locus of care" in the community.[8] Community mental health nursing emerged within the context of the mental hygiene movement. This movement arose in the 1920s and 1930s in response to concerns about the deplorable state of asylums and eugenic concerns about the mental health of the population, in relation to immigration, class and race-based fears of degeneration, and purported uncivilized behavior and an alleged digressing morality of the lower classes.[9] Both in the United States and Canada national philanthropic committees for mental hygiene were formed during this time and an international federation was founded in 1924.[10] Psychiatrists and nurses engaged with public mental health in response to initiatives of these national committees. While it was difficult for nurses to carve out roles in prevention and outpatient work because of nurses' firm tie to the institutions, they did so nevertheless, influencing the incorporation of mental health nursing in home and school visiting and in "after-care" following discharge into nursing thought and practice. The "new" community care in 1970s seems a continuation of some of these professional roles first envisioned during the mental hygiene movement and the emergence of social psychiatry, a development that transgressed national boundaries.[11] In the US, Church[12] addressed the development of community mental health nursing in the US after the passage of the National Mental Health Act in 1946 until the 1960s, but she did not exam-

---

8   Boschma/Mychajlunow/Yonge (2005); Dooley (2004); Hicks (2011); Thifault (2009); Tipliski (2004).
9   Dyck (2013); MacLennan (1987); Pols (1997); Sillars (1983).
10 Roland (1990); Thomson (1995).
11 Boschma (2012); Brouns (2010); Church (1987); Dyck (2011).
12 Church (1987).

ine the evolution of community-based care after 1960. In Canada, Sillars[13] looked at the history of community mental health nursing in Toronto prior to the 1950s. She found that as their fields professionalized, social workers and psychologist assumed much of this work rather than nurses.

Only few studies have focused on community care in the post-1950s time period. Focusing on psychiatric nursing in the UK, Nolan[14] noted that the National Health Service in 1948 prompted a shift towards outpatient and community care as did a new mental health act in 1959. Large numbers of long term hospitalized patients were discharged from mental hospitals, but specialized training in community care for nurses was not implemented until the 1970s with new roles for community psychiatric nurses. In Canada, where psychiatric nursing as a distinct professional field developed only in the western provinces, the title community psychiatric nursing was first established in the province of Saskatchewan in the post-1950s era.[15] The election of the Co-operative Commonwealth Federation government in 1944 in Saskatchewan triggered many new health reforms, including a public health insurance plan in the late 1940s. A strong emphasis was placed on the improvement of mental hospitals and its staff, including expansion and improvement of psychiatric nursing education.[16] Martin[17] observed how the Saskatchewan government passed an early deinstitutionalization policy, called the Saskatchewan Plan, which had a unique influence on the education and professional identity of psychiatric nurses. The mental health service officers approved of a new community-based role for the many nurses who suddenly found themselves in oversupply because of a massive move of patients out of mental hospitals hospital. No structure was in place to address some of the complex problems this move created. In the 1960s, the Saskatchewan government formally designed a new Community Psychiatric Nursing role.[18] Planned more or less as an afterthought, these nurses began to provide follow-up care for discharged persons from the mental hospitals, while formerly hospital-based psychiatric nursing education moved from the Psychiatric Services Branch to the Department of Education in 1972. Soon psychiatric nurses in other western Canadian mental hospitals followed this pattern.[19] In Alberta, graduates of hospital-based psychiatric nursing programs importantly contributed to the renewal of institutional nursing practice during the 1960s and 1970s, while some, similar to patterns in Saskatchewan, engaged with new work in the community to accommodate and follow discharged patients.[20] Interestingly, in BC, the RH hospital-based school of psychiatric nursing also discontinued in 1972 and the

13   Sillars (1983).
14   Nolan (1993).
15   Hicks (2011); Martin (2003).
16   Dyck (2008); Hicks (2011); Tipliski (2004).
17   Martin (2003).
18   Martin (2003).
19   Boschma/Mychajlunow/Yonge (2005).
20   Boschma (2012); Boschma/Mychajlunow/Yonge (2005).

program transferred to the Department of Education.[21] Yet, there is no record of BC developing a community-focused psychiatric nursing program at this time. The integration of psychiatric nurses in new community-based services often happened in an unplanned way – not as an integrated part of policy development. Still, a changing therapeutic climate and focus on rehabilitation within and "outside" mental hospitals changed the work and professional identity of nurses with a new community focus as the case example of Pioneer House suggests.

Patterns of downsizing mental hospitals differed from country to country – some countries shifted gears seemingly almost overnight, for example the United States and Italy, whereas others, such as the Netherlands, never really engaged with sweeping deinstitutionalization, in part because that country did not have large institutions to begin with, whereas in still others, such as Canada, deinstitutionalization was a prolonged process over several decades, with interprovincial differences, lasting sometimes into the 1990s.[22] But in all countries the public understanding, and hence, mental health policy changed. The large mental hospital and the farm-like rhythm it had followed fell into discredit – new social, medical, and therapeutic arrangements outside the confinement of a custodial institutional structure were developed based on new 20th century managerial and professional foundations.[23]

These new foundations of nursing work and organization of care intersected with other social changes in mental health service beginning in the mid-twentieth century: new perspectives on consumer voice and patient rights.[24] The poor circumstances in mental hospital became the target of counter-cultural activism and anti-psychiatric protest, arising in some countries as early as the 1950s, but spreading throughout the western world in the 1960s and 1970s.[25] Much of the critique centered on the legal and ethical constraints of forced confinement as well as on the hegemonic medical model that seemed to determine the power relationships in institutions. The call for patient autonomy and rehabilitative, community care and efforts to reduce stigma and social control were closely aligned. Patients became a new voice in the context of community-based care.

An articulate voice of patients was not an entirely new phenomenon in the 1970s. Although a historiography on patients is a relatively recent phenomenon, an autobiographical literature existed since the beginning of the century, and even before.[26] Notably, Beers'[27] biography had been at the heart of the mental hygiene movement. Whether it was on their experiences of

21 AR MHSB 1974, pp. L73.
22 Gijswijt-Hofstra/Oosterhuis/Vijselaar/Freeman (2005); Macfarlane/Fortin/Fox/Gundry/Oshry/Warren (1997); Sealy/Whitehead (2004).
23 Gijswijt-Hofstra/Oosterhuis/Vijselaar/Freeman (2005).
24 Tomes (2006); Hoffman/Tomes/Grob/Schlesinger (2011).
25 Chamberlain (1978); Crossley (2006); Foucault (1965); Goffman (1961); Hunsche (2008); Moran/Wright (2006); Scull (1979).
26 Davies (2001); Porter (1987); Reaume (2000).
27 Beers (1908).

illness or health care, or a critique of the system, patients have used both au-
tobiography and fiction to make their views known.[28] Political engagement,
cultural critique, and advocacy for change shaped an emerging historiography, including oral history and (auto)biographical studies on the place of the
patient in psychiatry post-1950s.[29] Media and film added to the populariza-
tion of the patient experience, a most influential and lasting example being
One Flew Over the Cuckoo's Nest – both the novel, published in 1962, and the
1975 film.[30]

In many places throughout Europe and North America, new collectives of
counter-cultural activism among patients and professionals alike, resulted in
new alternatives of community living.[31] To emphasize their political stance
and connection to the "mad- or liberation- movement," patients resisted their
identification with the medical model and many no longer identified as "patient." Being a "user of services" constituted one as a "consumer of services."
Similarly, having been subjected to psychiatric services perceived as harmful
constituted one as a "survivor" of them.[32] Critics, activists, and advocacy
groups joined forces with a broad group of protesters from many streams, including professionals, in an (international) legal campaign to reverse power in
psychiatry.[33]

The example of Pioneer House seems to support the importance of detailed analysis of grassroots initiatives in community care to better grasp how
people found new models and identities to accommodate to new models of
care. Because of its link with MPA members, the group around Pioneer House
was closely aligned with the new ideas drawn from the psychiatric liberation
or "mad" movement. Although much of the outward public protest faded
away by the late 1980s, by then patient advocates were well integrated into
many legal, professional, policy bodies, and advisory councils, well situated to
influence policy making.[34] Moreover, many consumers found new employment in mental health work and peer support.[35] An analysis of the day-to-day
realities of nurses' work highlights how the institutional context of care – with
all its dilemmas – had to be renegotiated and reinvented when services
"moved" into the community. Very little nursing history research includes the
experience and contribution of patients towards these changes in service. The
analysis of the early foundation of Pioneer House highlights how nurses
worked closely with patients and – a largely overlooked category – volunteers.
The latter group formed an essential new influence in post-1950s mental
health care.

28   Beamish (2003); Chamberlain (1978); Davies (2001); Shimrat (1997).
29   Baur (2011); Ingram (2005); Kerr (2003).
30   Kesey (1962); Hirshbein/Sarvananda (2008).
31   Burstow/Weitz (1988); Chamberlain (1978); Crossley (2006); Harrington (2008); Morri-
     son (2005).
32   Shimrat (1997); Tomes (2006).
33   Crossley (2006).
34   Everett (2000); Hoffman/Tomes/Grob/Schlesinger (2011); Shimrat (1997).
35   Boschma/Davies/Morrow (2014).

Background

In the remainder, I will first provide some background on the way the mental hospital already had begun to change from the 1950s onwards, which contributed to the context of change that made the establishment of Pioneer House possible. Then I examine the development of Pioneer House itself. In Canada, beginning in the late 1940s and 1950s several factors enhanced downsizing of large mental hospitals: increased public funding for health care as a result of post second world war economic prosperity, new entitlement to health as a right, rapid expansion of general hospital care, and new professional confidence in the use of new psychotropic medication beginning in the early 1950s. More patients left the mental hospitals, disrupting established patterns of long-term admission of people with mental illness. All parties involved seemed to scramble to accommodate a growing number of short-term admissions to the mental hospitals and to new outpatient and general hospital psychiatric services. Moreover, a growing number of elderly and mentally disabled people were discharged into the community or transferred to other institutions, a process also framed as transinstitutionalization.[36]

The Riverview provincial mental hospital – located in Coquitlam, had been in existence since the early 20th century. From the outset, it continuously expanded its service and building complex.[37] From the 1950s onwards, however, this hospital began to drastically reduce its number of patients and gradually developed a more outward looking focus, seeking more active engagements with the surrounding community.[38] Whereas in some countries mental hospitals closed in the 1960s, Canada had a prolonged process of deinstitutionalization and mental hospital downsizing. BC's Riverview hospital only recently closed.[39]

In BC, first governmental initiatives to accommodate more patients outside "the walls" of the mental hospital took in BC the form of a Boarding Home program, which built upon existing welfare legislation and collaboration between the mental health branch and the welfare department by placing discharged patients in boarding homes originally set up for indigent elderly and other poverty-stricken dependents of the state.[40] When medically oriented, publicly funded accommodation such as nursing homes were established in the mid-20th century these older "old age" homes obtained a new purpose. This strategy proved to be ineffective, however, when in the 1970s massive numbers of former psychiatric patients had to find places to live in the community.

36 Boschma (2011); Hector (2001); Ostry (2009).
37 Thompson (1972).
38 Tucker (1971).
39 Boschma (2011).
40 Booth (1961); Crum/Jamieson (1972).

Until the mid-1970s there was considerable federal funding in Canada to improve the mental hospitals, for example through a national health grants program, but there was little thought about enduring support in community living for people with mental illness outside the hospital, nor about a need for nurses following discharged patients.[41] The problem was that for the ever growing number of discharged patients neither facilities nor support for community living existed. Changing this conundrum was a core motivation of the psychiatric nurses, volunteers, and consumers at RH in joining forces to found the RHVA. I will briefly discuss each of the three founding groups.

Psychiatric Nurses at RH

The BC Mental Health Services Branch had established a School for Psychiatric Nurses at RH in 1930 to enhance the quality of its staff and to attract more nurses to staff the wards. In 1950, when the mental hospital patient population was at its peak, and the Branch shifted direction, the need for more trained personnel became even more prominent. Introduction of psychotropic medication, short-term treatment and early discharge actually increased admission. More "active treatment", and the effort to turn the hospital into a "therapeutic community" placed further demands on personnel.[42] Health care personnel were in short supply throughout the 1950s. Psychiatrists were hard to attract as were social workers, occupational therapists and clinical psychologists, but the most desperate need was for nurses. Supply of nurses never seemed to keep up with demand. The School kept being enlarged to accommodate more student nurses, and large numbers of psychiatric aides were hired during the 1950s and 1960s to fill the gaps.[43]

On the hospital grounds, and in the wards, however, this shortage of staff translated into a relatively high level of control for psychiatric nurses over daily ward routines and day-to-day management of patients albeit with little support to introduce change. Most prominent therapeutic changes on the wards during the 1950s and 1960s were the *opening* of the wards and gender unitization. In order to normalize hospital culture, influenced by wider social changes – men and women were "unitized" onto the same wards, and placed in a "group living" situation. Patients obtained more freedom, being permitted to walk freely on the grounds or in small groups with "ground-privileges" supervised by a nurse. Nurses were mainly learning from each other through experience, from the few nurses who did receive some advanced education, and from helpful psychologists and social workers. To enhance so-called "active treatment" RH opened a large new Recreation Hall with an auditorium,

---

41 Boschma/Haynes/Gorrie (2012).
42 AR MHSB 1956, pp. Q59–63; Jones (1953).
43 Information on the RH School of Psychiatric Nurses is drawn from the Annual Reports of the Mental Health Services Branch of British Columbia – Reports on the School of Nursing (AR MHSB, 1951–74).

a gymnasium, a cafeteria, and a large bowling alley, giving patients (and staff) access to films, dances, sports, bowling – all within walking distance. A capable group of patients soon helped in the organization of recreational activities.[44]

On the wards, nurses became coordinators of all this new work.[45] They started social groups, oversaw the introduction of patient ward councils, and helped men and women adjust to co-ed living. Because of their medical skills, they also administered and monitored the new psychotropic medication introduced from the 1950s onwards. The coordination of patients' living, work and recreational activities on the wards basically rested with the nursing staff. As efforts to discharge more patients in the community grew, initially mainly through a boarding house program still closely connected to the hospital, some nurses found employ in new community work.[46] But the overall focus was on improving the existing context of institutional care and adapting to the growing volume of shorter-term admissions *in* the hospital.[47]

Volunteers

At RH, the involvement of volunteer-citizens in mental health work began in the 1950s. Volunteer involvement was an important influence on the shift in the landscape of mental health care from the 1950s onwards.[48] In 1952, the Canadian Mental Health Association (CMHA), a voluntary group aiming to enhance public awareness, reduce stigma, and normalize mental illness, opened a BC Division at the Riverview hospital.[49] Many of their member volunteers were non-working women with time on their hands. The CMHA's main purpose was to develop a public mental health strategy to reduce public fears and increase awareness of mental illness.[50] In collaboration with RH the BC Division set up a Volunteer Department in 1955. While the CMHA recruited, screened and trained the volunteers, nursing staff helped to coordinate this new volunteer work, facilitating volunteer visits on the wards and guiding new volunteer activities. The CMHA volunteers started an Apparel shop, for example, on the hospital grounds where patients could now "shop" for non-institutional clothes and they ran in-hospital visiting programs, while also helping with recreational activities. However, somewhat contradictory to the original goals, these volunteers became an enduring part of the *hospital community*. Their help was most welcomed by nurses who – always short staffed – could use any help. By 1973, registered nurse Sydney Baird, then

---

44   AR MHSB 1967, pp. G47–8; Coppard (1963).
45   AR MHSB 1955, pp. M99; AR MHSB 1967, pp. G57–8.
46   Interview Dewar (2009).
47   Boschma (2011).
48   Mooney/Reinarz (2009); Whyte (2011).
49   Baird (1974); CMHA (1960).
50   CMHA (1960).

appointed coordinator of Volunteer Services, proudly reported that, "over 300 dedicated volunteers" donated their services – for which "their reward is satisfaction", while "their service is invaluable".[51] Unpaid volunteer work had become an integral part of the hospital organization.

While these services greatly enhanced life *in* the hospital, barriers for people with mental illness to transition out of the hospital and live in the community continued to be high and attracted increasing public attention. Public outcry over poor mental hospital care and lack of community resources grew. Mental patients also became more visible in the community when they began to be discharged in larger numbers. As of the 1960s, the BC government had begun discharging long-term mentally ill people into the community by placing them in so-called Boarding Homes: a model that in reality proved limited. Psychiatric nurse Carol Ann Russell remembered:

> I saw some of it happening in the '70s, [...] at RH, [...] there was a big move to [...] put people into the community. [It seemed great but] [...] in reality that wasn't great. [...] [clients], were leaving RH, they were coming into the community and they were [...] sitting in some living room in a [boarding] house somewhere. They [...] had a more integrated community life at Riverview where there was the store and the movies and the bowling [...] When they came to the community, which was supposedly a better deal for them, there was no infrastructure in place to help integrate these people into the community. [They] were less active than they had been at Riverview.[52]

They also often returned.

Patients (consumers)

The push to broaden volunteer work at RH into a new outward direction, and attracting nurses to engage with this work *in* the community came from a new group of "volunteers" emerging in the 1970s: Consumers or ex-patients who had organized themselves into the MPA. Part of the larger anti-psychiatric movement, they had profound critique of the established medical model of psychiatry, and an interest in patient rights. The MPA focused attention on the lack of resources outside of the institution and organized themselves in a patient-run organization. Within a year or so they ran several communal homes in Vancouver, a drop-in centre and published a monthly newsletter, *In a Nutshell*, while, in 1973, they began to visit their peers in RH and new general hospital psychiatric departments in the area on a weekly basis.[53] Their ideal of community living was based on the principles they felt were important: friendship and understanding. They also radicalized matters on the hospital grounds. They wanted more radical change and reverse power structures. And so they did. Dave Beamish, for example, was the initiator of the MPA Riverview extension program. He had become MPA member in the early

---

51   Baird (1974), pp. 11–2.
52   Interview Russell (2009).
53   Beamish (1973). See also MPA Founders Collective (2013).

1970s, finding a welcome home in the MPA community when he was desperate to leave the boarding home at which he initially had ended up after being discharged from RH.[54] The MPA experience was transforming for him. He not only found community, but also developed skill as employed coordinator at one of the MPA residential homes and found creative space to engage in writing poetry.[55] He became involved with the weekly visiting program at MPA, visiting the wards at RH on a regular basis to provide patients with information and support – a political act as much as one of offering peer support. Starting the MPA Riverview extension program was part of the ongoing presence of MPA at RH. Among other initiatives to assert a strong patient voice, the MPA triggered a new patient-led council at RH and ensured themselves a permanent MPA office in the Volunteer Department.[56]

Nurses *and* patients drew on their experience within the institution *and* on their engagement with an emerging, radicalized patient movement in organizing this new form of care. The way nurses' work with patients, their craft, had already changed in the hospital prior to the 1970s, and had generated new experiential knowledge, explains in part the way they engaged with community care. In tandem, in part drawing on their hospital experience, ex-patients paved new ways in building enduring support for vulnerable people.

Pioneer House

Oral history interviews with Colleen Dewar and Carol Ann Russell – two psychiatric nurses who had started their nursing education at RH in 1967 and 1969 respectively, and were involved with Pioneer House from the start, and an interview with Dave Beamish, former RH patient and MPA member, allowed an intimate understanding of the way the RHVA initiated Pioneer House. As said, David Beamish was an instrumental leader in this change. In developing his role at RH he had a close ally in Fran Phillips, a former public health nurse, who he knew from MPA – in the 1970s, she had joined the MPA as an ally and Residence Coordinator.[57] Politically minded, neither Beamish nor Phillips liked staff-driven models of care – they wanted more patient control and believed in a self-help philosophy. The politicized MPA group found the pragmatically oriented RH volunteers and psychiatric nurses who ran the Volunteer Department on their side, and together they formed the new RHVA. Colleen Dewar, an experienced psychiatric nurse interested in new opportunities in community care, was hired by the board in 1982 to set up the home and the first patients moved in in 1983.[58] That year another psychiatric nurse from RH, Carol Ann Russell, also joined the staff, while Beamish be-

---

54 Interview Beamish (2010, 2011).
55 Beamish (1976, 2003); Interview Beamish (2010; 2011).
56 Task Committee on Proposed Patients' Council, RH (1979).
57 Interview Beamish (2011), Phillips (1976).
58 Interview Dewar (2009), "Pioneer House to Open Soon" (1982).

came senior worker. In setting up Pioneer House, they took example from the
MPA model of communal living in setting up a first home, Pioneer House.
Beamish recalled how they had to familiarize the staff with the self-help philosophy the MPA valued: "Well, we had to train the staff [of Pioneer House]
because no-one, nobody had done that kind of work before."[59] The RHVA
board hired Phillips to direct their first initiative. Pioneer House markedly
differed from the existing boarding home model. Russell remembered Beamish as "someone who […] had been in the system, [and] this is what he felt was
needed […]. A lot of [what we did] was based on his personal experiences of
being a mental patient in the system in those days – and where he saw the
gaps."[60] These close personal and professional ties within the group generated
a new way of running the home *with* the residents – they all helped in the
work of the house – and it emerged as a grassroots process. Beamish recalled
that "We […] used to have a resident's meeting every week, I organized that."[61]

   While Phillips and Beamish clearly brought their activist MPA experience
to Pioneer House, Dewar and Russell appeared to have joined for more pragmatic reasons such as the hours and increased flexibility the work allowed
which permitted them to combine their position with their family responsibilities. They further appreciated the relative independence community work
provided and were attracted to the non-profit model because of the greater
independence it gave them. As Russell noted:

> I feel working in a non-profit organization, you can institute changes […] modify pro-
> grams […] without the bureaucracy, and although […] we were being paid considerably
> less than what the hospital were paying their nurses […] [which made it a hard decision],
> I'm a single parent […] but I was able to get the flexibility I needed […] with the satisfac-
> tion I was getting from the work […] I just decided to stay here.[62]

In the first year she was hired, Dewar prepared the location and arranged the
licensing requirements for Pioneer House. There was no psychologist involved, nor a social worker. Dewar arranged for a consulting physician with
whom she set up a system for medication management –, a licensing requirement. She found a cook, a bookkeeper and a nutritionist for the same reason,
but otherwise the place was run by nurses and former patients. Indeed a profound power-reversal if compared to the hierarchical institutional structure of
RH. Perhaps because of her more pragmatic lens, Dewar was able to navigate
Pioneer House through many bureaucratic obstacles. For example, she introduced the first community self-medication program, skillfully negotiating the
bureaucratic licensing regulations: "We started the first self-medication program. I had to write to Victoria (the BC capital) to receive permission for that.
So we started that and we have a module and now in every program we have,
we have a graduated self-medication program."[63]

---

59   Interview Beamish (2011).
60   Interview Russell (2009).
61   Interview Beamish (2011).
62   Interview Russell (2009).
63   Interview Dewar (2009).

As can be imagined, Pioneer House was not without its new dilemmas as staff sought to find a balance between self-help, care, control and patient involvement. Soon internal discords centered on the question what kind of work projects would best fit the needs of the residents. Phillips for example promoted self-sufficiency and started a catering business. Yet, the board and other nurses soon felt such a project was unsustainable.[64] Nurses had to do most of the work which ran against the goal of patient self-determination.

Tension also rose over funding, particularly once the provincial government increased its control over community agencies by subsidizing the cost of running the facilities. Up until the mid-1980s staff had been able to independently decide who would live at Pioneer House. But during that time the provincial government began to assert more control over residential community services, as they now were called, both in terms of funding and placement policies, through its local mental health services and the appointment of a placement coordinator at a Mental Health Centre (MHC) established in New Westminster.[65] Pioneer House was part of that jurisdiction. Phillips and Beamish deeply resented such control, preferring to decide who could live in the house for themselves, and were ill-prepared to accept MHC input.[66] For them, the MHC resembled governmental bureaucracy and seemed only an exponent of medical and bureaucratic control. Complete self-control by patients and staff over who could live in the house ran, in the end, against increasing governmental control over admission in community-run facilities. In the late 1980s the home ran the risk of losing their funding if they would not accept some government-imposed regulation of admission. The radical, founding approach "was a little too rough around the edges, in retrospect," Russell noted. We "really, really needed to change the relationship that we had with the [provincial government services] because let's face it, they were contracting our service," she pointed out.[67] To her, and the RHVA board, accepting a certain level of governmental control would not overrule a democratic, consumer-driven ideal of rehabilitative services, but rather be a strategic effort to protect the model's rehabilitative principles in the face of continuously shifting pressures of bureaucratic control and funding. They seemed to accept it as a necessary compromise while Phillips left.

It could be argued that the shift to community care was not a radical break with an institutional context and service but rather a renegotiation of power and control of them. Both groups, nurses and patients, drew from their institutional experience, built on alignments formed within an institutional context, and negotiated control and connections in the community. While building new community connections and services, nurses and patients accommodated to different views around the parameters of care and rehabilita-

---

64   Interview Dewar (2009).
65   Mental Health Services, BC Ministry of Health, Annual Report 1981, Victoria BC, pp. 90–91.
66   Interview Beamish (2011).
67   Interview Russell (2009).

tion, the inevitable compliance with bureaucratic control, and ultimately about the balance between the two – not unlike their predecessors in the institution also had done.

Conclusion

The new RHVA brought together patients, volunteers and nurses on the grounds of the provincial mental hospital in BC, to join forces in creating a new facility for community living. Former patients who moved into the new Pioneer House found a staff supporting them to take their own decisions, do their own planning, and construct community in a new way. As said, Beamish and his MPA-ally Phillips had an essential role spreading the MPA model at RH. The RHVA also included two very different generations of volunteers, 1950s and 1960s married women and some men who engaged in volunteer work out of humanitarian motives but also still grounded in deeply patriarchal hierarchies not unlike the nurses, and a next wave of volunteer work at the hospital stemming from new more radical 1960s and 1970s philosophies which questioned patriarchal and authoritarian relationships giving voice to patient interests in new ways. Nurses, in new roles of community psychiatric nurse, became caught up in this transformation as well. Moreover, patient engagement with mental health work made existing boundaries between professional and patient work more fluid and negotiable. The example of Pioneer House also highlights how dilemmas of care versus control that had played out in institutional care were reproduced when shifting to community services. As the RHVA navigated the power relationships within the group under the constraints of a certain level of bureaucratic control, they in fact accommodated to such control in order to sustain a model of community living that was the larger interest of the RHVA. In this endeavor patients not only carved out a more prominent role in caring work, the collaborative initiative also interrupted established perceptions of both practitioners and patients in mental health.

Bibliography

Archival sources

Private collection Geertje Boschma

Interview with Dave Beamish by Megan Davies, Vancouver, June 2010.
Interview with Dave Beamish by author, Vancouver, August 2011.
Interview with Colleen Dewar by author, New Westminster, February 2009.
Interview with Carol Ann Russell by Nerrisa Bonifacio, New Westminster, August 2009.

Electronic sources

MPA Founders Collective: The inmates are running the asylum: Stories from the MPA [Mental Patient Association]. A documentary about the group that transformed Canada's psychiatric landscape. DVD, 36-minutes. Producer: Megan Davies; Co-Producer: Marina Morrow; Associate Co-Producer: Geertje Boschma. © History of Madness Productions 2013. http://historyofmadness.ca/the-inmates-are-running-the-asylum/

Printed sources

Annual Report (AR) Mental Health Services Branch of British Columbia (MHSB), Victoria BC (1951–1974).
Baird, Sydney: Riverview's Volunteer Activities – 1973. In: Newsletter, [BC] Mental Health Branch, Department of Health Services and Hospital Insurance, March (1974), pp. 11–2.
Beamish, Dave: Hospital Visiting. In: In a Nutshell. The MPA Newsletter, 2(1) (1973), pp. 5.
Beamish, Dave: MPA Riverview Extension Program. In: In a Nutshell. The MPA Newsletter, 4(4) (1976), pp. 5.
Beers, Clifford: A Mind That Found Itself. Pittsburg 1908.
CMHA (Canadian Mental Health Association): Milestones in Mental Health: A Record of Achievements … the Canadian Mental Health Association 1918–1958. Toronto 1960.
Coppard, A. E: Rehabilitation Programme (Staff Publication), British Columbia / Riverview Hospital 1963.
Mental Health Services – BC Ministry of Health, Annual Report, 1981, Victoria BC 1981.
Pioneer House to Open Soon Under Riverview Volunteers: In: Insight, Riverview Hospital Newsletter 1(8) February (1982), pp.1.
Phillips, Fran. MPA Residence Program: In Memoriam. In: In a Nutshell. The Mental Patients Association Newsletter 4(2) (1976), pp. 12.
Task Committee on Proposed Patients' Council, RH. (1979) "Terms of Reference for a Patients' Council at Riverview Hospital," Draft Proposal of the Task Committee on Proposed Patients' Council, RH. Document collection, Riverview Hospital Historical Society.
Thompson, Robert. H.: A Summary of the Growth and Development of Mental Health Facilities in British Columbia, 1850–1970. BC Mental Health Branch, BC Government 1972.

Secondary research literature

Baur, Nicole: On Site: Oral Testimonies in Mental Health History. In: Social History of Medicine 24 (2011), 2, pp. 484–487.
Beamish, Dave: King of the World, Poems and Prose (Chapbook), Vancouver 2003.
Booth, Beatrice: Family Care Homes for Mental Patients. Unpublished thesis. University of British Columbia 1961.
Boschma, Geertje: Deinstitutionalization Reconsidered: Geographic and Demographic Changes in Mental Health Care in British Columbia and Alberta, 1950–1980. In: Histoire Sociale / Social History 44 (2011), 88, pp. 223–256.
Boschma, Geertje: Community Mental Health Nursing in Alberta, Canada: An Oral History. In: Nursing History Review 20 (2012), pp. 103–135.
Boschma, Geertje; Yonge, Olive; Mychajlunow, Lorraine: Gender and Professional Identity in Psychiatric Nursing Practice in Alberta, Canada, 1930–1975. In: Nursing Inquiry 12 (2005), 4, pp. 243–55.

Boschma, Geertje; Haney, Catherine; Gorrie, Margaret: Gender, Work, and Identity: Consumer Perspectives on Rehabilitation and Recovery in Mental Health Care. In: The Bulletin of the UK Association for the History of Nursing 1 (2012), 1, pp. 8–19.

Boschma, Geertje; Davies, Megan; Morrow, Marine: Those People Known as Mental Patients: Professional and Patient Engagement in Community Mental Health n Vancouver, BC in the 1970s. In: Oral History Forum / d'histoire orale 34 (2014) [Electronic journal: http://www.oralhistoryforum.ca/index.php/ohf/issue/current]

Brouns, Ger: Social-psychiatrische verpleegkunde: de ontwikkeling van een verpleegkundig specialisme in het domein van de Nederlandse sociale psychiatrie [Social-psychiatric nursing: The development of a nursing specialty in the domain of Dutch social psychiatry]. Unpublished dissertation. Universiteit Maastricht 2010.

Burstow, Bonnie; Weitz, Don (eds.): Shrink Resistant: The Struggle against Psychiatry in Canada. Vancouver 1988.

Chamberlain, Judi: On Our Own: Patient-Controlled Alternatives to the Mental Health System. New York 1978.

Church, Olga: From Custody to Community in Psychiatric Nursing. In: Nursing Research 36 (1978), 1, pp. 48–55.

Crossley Nick: Contesting Psychiatry: Social Movements in Mental Health. New York 2006.

Crum, M.; Jamieson, J: An Analysis of the British Columbia Regional Boarding Home Programme. Unpublished thesis. University of British Columbia 1972.

Davies, Kerry: Silent and Censured Travelers? Patients' Narratives and Patients' Voices: Perspectives on the History of Mental Illness since 1948. In: Social History of Medicine 14 (2001), 2, pp. 267–292.

Dooley, Chris: They Gave Their Care, but We Gave Loving Care: Defining and Defending Boundaries of Skill and Craft in the Nursing Service of a Manitoba Mental Hospital during the Great Depression. In: Canadian Bulletin of Medical History 21 (2004), 2, pp. 229–251.

Dyck, Erika: Psychedelic Psychiatry: LSD from Clinic to Campus. Baltimore 2008.

Dyck, Erika: Dismantling the Asylum and Charting New Pathways into the Community: Mental Health Care in Twentieth Century Canada. In: Histoire Sociale / Social History 44 (2011), 88, pp. 181–196.

Dyck, Erika: Facing Eugenics: Reproduction, Sterilization and the Politics of Choice. Toronto 2013.

Everett, Barbara: A Fragile Revolution: Consumers and Psychiatric Survivors Confront the Power of the Mental Health System. Waterloo 2000.

Foucault, Michel: Madness and Civilization. New York 1965.

Gijswijt-Hofstra, Marijke; Oosterhuis, Harry; Vijselaar, Joost; Hugh Freeman (eds.): Psychiatric Cultures Compared: Psychiatry and Mental Health Care in the Twentieth Century. Amsterdam 2005.

Goffman, Erving: Asylums: Essays on the Condition of the Social Situation of Mental Patients and Other Inmates. New York 1961.

Harrington, Valerie: Voices beyond the Asylum: A Post-War History of Mental Health Services in Manchester and Salford. Unpublished dissertation. University of Manchester 2008.

Hector, Ian: Changing Funding Patterns and the Effect on Mental Health Care in Canada. In: Rae-Grant, Quentin (ed.): Psychiatry in Canada: 50 Years, 1951–2001. Ottawa 2001, pp. 59–76.

Hicks, Beverly: Gender, Politics, and Regionalism: Factors in the Evolution of Registered Psychiatric Nursing in Manitoba, 1920–1960. In: Nursing History Review 19 (2011), pp. 103–126.

Hirshbein, Laurie; Sarvananda, Sharmalie: History, Power, and Electricity: American Popular Magazine Accounts Of Electroconvulsive Therapy, 1940–2005. In: Journal of the History of the Behavioral Sciences 44 (2008), 1, pp. 1–18.

Hoffman, Beatrix; Tomes, Nancy; Grob, Rachel; Schlesinger, Mark (eds.): Patients as Policy Actors. New Jersey 2011.

Hunsche, Petra: De strijdbare patient: Van Gekkenbeweging to Cliënten Bewustzijn – Portretten 1970–2000 [The Fighting Spirited Patient: From Mad-Movement to Client (or Consumer) Consciousness – Portraits 1970–2000]. Amsterdam 2008.

Ingram, Richard: Troubled Being and Being Troubled: Subjectivity in the Light of Problems of the Mind. Unpublished dissertation. University of British Columbia 2005.

Jones, Maxwell: The Therapeutic Community: A New Treatment Method in Psychiatry. New York 1953.

Kerr, David: "We Know What the Problem is": Using Oral History to Develop a Collaborative Analysis of Homelessness from the Bottom Up. In: The Oral History Review 30 (2003), 1, pp. 27–45.

Kesey, Kevin: One Flew Over the Cuckoo's Nest. New York 1962.

Macfarlane, D., Fortin, P., Fox, J., Gundry, S., Oshry, J. and Warren, E.: Clinical and Human Resource Planning for the Downsizing of Psychiatric Hospitals: The British Columbia Experience. In: Psychiatric Quarterly 68 (1997), 1, pp. 25–42.

MacLennan, David: Beyond the Asylum: Professionalization and the Mental Hygiene Movement in Canada, 1914–1928. In: Canadian Bulletin of Medical History 4 (1987), pp. 7–23.

Martin, Angela: Determinants of Destiny: The Professional Development of Psychiatric Nurses in Saskatchewan. Unpublished thesis, University of Regina 2003.

Mooney, Graham; Reinarz, Jonathan (eds.): Permeable Walls: Historical Perspectives on Hospital and Asylum Visiting. Amsterdam 2009.

Moran, James; Wright, David (eds.): Mental Health and Canadian Society: Historical Perspectives. Montreal 2006.

Morrison, Linda: Talking Back to Psychiatry. The Consumer/Survivor/Ex-Patient Movement. London 2005.

Nolan, Peter: A History of Mental Health Nursing. London 1993.

Ostry, Aleck: The Foundations of National Public Hospital Insurance. In: Canadian Bulletin of Medical History 26 (2009), 2, pp. 261–82.

Pols, Johannes: Managing the Mind: The Culture of American Mental Hygiene, 1910–1950. Unpublished dissertation. University of Pennsylvania 1997.

Porter, Roy: A Social History of Madness. London 1987.

Reaume, Geoffrey: Remembrance of Patients Past: Patient Life at the Toronto Hospital for the Insane, 1870–1940. Ontario 2000.

Roland, Charles G.: Clarence Hincks: Mental Health Crusader. Toronto 1990.

Scull, Andrew: Museums of Madness: The Social Organization of Insanity in Nineteenth-Century England. London 1979.

Sealy, Patricia; Whitehead, Paul C.: Forty Years of Deinstitutionalization of Psychiatric Services in Canada: An Empirical Assessment. In: Canadian Journal of Psychiatry 49 (2004), pp. 249–257.

Shimrat, Irit: Call Me Crazy: Stories from the Mad Movement. Vancouver 1997.

Sillars, Dorothy: The Development of Community Mental Health Nursing in Toronto from 1917–1947. Unpublished thesis, University of Toronto, 1983.

Thifault, Marie-Claude: Au-Delà d'un Role de Protection à l'Égard des Aliénés: Initiation à l'Art du Nursing à l'Hôpital Saint-Jean-de-Dieu, 1912–1915. In: S. Yaya (ed.) Pouvoir Médical et Santé Totalitaire: Conséquences Socio-Anthropologiques et Éthiques. Québec 2009, pp. 341–358.

Thomson, Mathew: Mental Hygiene as an International Movement. In: Weindling, Paul (ed.): International Health Organizations and Movements, 1918–1939. Cambridge 1995, pp. 283–304.

Tipliski, Veryl M.: Parting at the crossroads: The Emergence of Education for Psychiatric Nursing in three Canadian Provinces, 1909–1955. In: Canadian Bulletin of Medical History 21 (2004), 2, pp. 253–279.

Tomes, Nancy: The Patient as a Policy Factor: A Historical Case Study of the Consumer/
    Survivor Movement in Mental Health. In: Health Affairs 25 (2006), pp. 720–729.
Tucker, Frederick G.: Mental Health Services in British Columbia. In: Canada's Mental
    Health 19 (1971), 6, pp. 7–12.
Whyte, Jayne: Visiting the Mentally Ill: Volunteer Visitors at Saskatchewan Hospital, Wey-
    burn 1950–1965. In: Histoire Sociale / Social History 44 (2011), 88, pp. 289–304.

Nurses, Patients and Their Families

Configurations of Dispute – Everyday Lives of Nurses and Patients in an Asylum at the Turn of the Century

Jens Gründler

Summary

This article focuses on the relationship between nurses and attendants and patients of one Scottish asylum at the turn of the 19th century. Taking case files and administrative sources it argues that the files tell a story of daily life in the institution that focuses on conflict and dispute. This highly symbolic image shaped the contemporaries' and historians' notion of asylum routines alike. Analysing the silence of the case files provides a completely different story of everyday life. The silence shows that daily routines were characterised by cooperation and tranquility. This impression is supported by patients' ego-documents that mention the relations between staff and patients. Cases of conflict in these documents feature as rare punctual differences in an otherwise peaceful coexistence based on mutual understanding and appreciation.

Introduction

At least since Erving Goffman's[1] analysis of asylums from mid-twentieth century it is widely accepted academic knowledge, that nurses and patients were closely intertwined. Nurses and attendants did the everyday work with patients.[2] They had to follow orders of the doctors while taxing and assessing the wishes and feelings of the patients. Being first "responders" their information structured and instructed the medical opinion of the physicians. Their position was sitting between a rock and a hard place and that did not change during the period under review here, that is around the turn of the 19th century. Even when they were professionally educated and trained as mental nurses from the 1890s onwards, they were still subjected to directives they had to follow strictly. Nevertheless, as Goffman has pointed out already, the staff had some room to negotiate with patients and manoeuvre around orders and standing orders in institutions, especially in large scale institutions.

Nurses and attendants in psychiatric hospitals, in Britain called asylums until about 1900 and then mental hospitals, have been under research for some decades. But while early research focused on professionalization of nurses,[3] in the last decades the perspective was extended on historical processes and developments as well as the practical side of everyday life in the

---

1 Goffman (1961).
2 The history of nursing has been a topic of research for the last decades. For introductions and overview of everyday working life and practices see Braunschweig (2006); D'Antonio (1999) or D'Antonio/Fairman/Whelan (2013). For a detailed overview of nursing history / care history in a German perspective see Christians/Kramer (2014).
3 See for example Nolan (1998).

asylum.[4] These analyses of practices in everyday life often focused of power relations within the doctor-patient-nurse triangle and violent conduct. Contemporaries as well as today's researchers described life in the asylums as brute and often dreary, accounting the patients and staff as antagonistic actors. The daily routines seemed to have been very conflictive, often resulting in physical violence and/or abuse, as historiographies have underlined. A recent example is Louise Hide's analysis of two London County Council Asylums at the turn of the century.[5] I would like to question this view on everyday life in asylums and instead point to the ambivalence of order and chaos, silence and noise. In asylums, both ends of the respective spectra – deafening noise and dead silence/complete chaos and shipshape order – were seldom occurrences. But while the case files often direct our understanding of the relationship of nursing staff and patients to chaos, noise and violence, different readings of these documents seem to be self-evident. Within this chapter I will try to give an answer to the question what we can learn about the relationship of patients and nursing staff from case files and patients' ego-documents. Taking 500 case files from Barony Pauper Lunatic Asylum Woodilee, the contemporary short form was Woodilee Asylum, including letters and notes of patients, administrative asylum sources, like letters by the superintendent to families and monthly reports[6], and parochial poor relief sources, like pauper case files and board minutes, this paper argues, that two narratives exist on everyday relationships between nurses and patients.[7] On the one hand, the case files tell a tale of two conflicting parties, putting the blame on patients' illnesses. The files seem to document that life in the asylum was violent, rowdyish, full of dispute and conflict. On the other hand, the silence of many files on clashes and unruly behaviour and the seldom mentioning of serious fighting at all tells another tale of life in the asylum without words: one of order, peace and calm. Taking those two sides into consideration, the paper will focus on the patients' perspectives on the relations between nursing staff and inmates, trying to establish whether or not different narratives of relations can be found and how the unfold.

The chapter is divided in four sections. Following this short introduction, the asylum as the place of the plot will be outlined in regard to size, therapeutic organization and outer fabric. Then, the focus is on the situation in regard to attendants' numbers, duties, social background and fluctuation. After that a more detailed view to relations between nurses and attendants on the one and

4   See for example Braunschweig (2006b) or Brimblecombe (2005).
5   Hide (2014).
6   In case of staff the only sources surviving in the archives are staff registers reaching from 1874 to 1978.
7   The chapter is based on my original research project on the connection of poverty and lunacy in Scotland from 1875 until the 1920s. The focus was put on the perspective of patients and their families during the process of admission, inpatient treatment and release as well as after release. Results were published in Gründler (2013).

patients on the other hand as noted in the patients' case files[8] will be provided. In a last step the focus is shifted on the patients' perspectives from letters and notes that were written by inmates and kept in the files.

Inner and outer fabric

Woodilee Asylum was erected and opened in the early 1870s. The first patients were admitted in October 1875 and the institution was the foremost lunatic asylum in Scotland in the eyes of its contemporaries. A local Glaswegian poor law authority financed it. Barony Parish, that authority, regularly checked and controlled the institution in financial and organizational matters. At the same time, the General Board of Commissioners for Lunacy in Scotland, the national administrative control, had to do visitations twice a year.

The asylum was built on the north western outskirts of Glasgow, adjoint to a railway line and close to a small train station. Also, it was only a 2.5 hours walk to central Glasgow. Therefore, access for visitors was extremely easy and quite cheap.

Being a modern farm asylum, in contemporary terms, the main form of treatment consisted in farm and workshop labour. James Rutherford, the first medical superintendent, worked with patients along the lines of moral treatment. Restraint and seclusion was rarely used, and a policy of open doors' was installed. There were usually no locked doors and only the head attendants and the medical staff had keys for certain doors inside the buildings. Accordingly, the grounds itself featured no walls or fences. Therefore the asylum was easily accessible for outsiders as well as patients could stroll off.[9]

8 Case files, as many historians have already stated, are a complicated source. This is not the place to discuss the source in detail. In the German context a controversy about the nature and contents of psychiatric case files has formed. Some historians – mainly of the field of medicine – argue, that the case files only allow insights into the medical case writing and the development of psychiatric science. See for example Ledebur (2011). In contrast, social historians (of medicine) are convinced that case files give insights into practices and routines, hierarchies and power and the relations between the different actors. See for example Andrews (1998); Nolte (2003); Gründler (2013). I am convinced medical case files can be used as source for social and cultural historians. Although they cannot share light into every detail of daily life in an institution, they can – for this chapter for example – give useful information for the analysis of the relations between nurses and attendants and patients.

9 "Mainly through fully occupying the patients, and thereby counteracting the tendency of manifestation of their insane ideas, it has been found practicable to carry out the open-door system of treatment. All the doors in the Asylum open with ordinary handles, and only the chief attendants are in possession of a key. I am not aware that this system is so fully carried out in any other large public Asylum. No untoward event has yet occurred to lead me to change my opinion, that by the diminution of apparent restrictions upon liberty, greater quietness and contentment are secured, which has its effect in promoting recovery and improvement. This is the first Asylum that has yet been erected without walled airing courts, and the want of them has never been felt to be a disadvantage. From the experience gained here, it is unlikely that any Asylum will now be built in Scotland

These regulations and the general therapeutic methods changed during the period under review. Especially with new Superintendents came new treatment policies. The first two Superintendents adhered to the regime of "moral treatment".[10] When Hamilton Marr took over in the 1890s he added much "science" to the therapies. The usage of pharmaceutical drugs and a more physical approach, gained ground. The case files seem to give a clear indication of the rising use of agents as Trional, Veronal and others. Especially within the first weeks after admission the sedation of patients is mentioned in much more files from the 1890s than before. Nevertheless, the character of the case files changed during that period as well. The staff noted much more information than in the decade and a half before. Again, the notes were particularly elaborate within the first weeks after admission. However, Hamilton Marr's more scientific approach could also be seen in the advancement of medical studies as well as in the drive to professionalize the staff through courses and certification. But the new therapeutic methods never replaced more traditional ways of treatment – work, rest and "moral treatment" were still used. Only in the late 1920s the outlook of the institution changed completely. Again, the change came in connection with a new superintendent. Henry Carre, then head of more than 2,000 patients, erected walls and fences and separated the institution from the outer world radically. The new Woodilee reminded visitors, staff and patients alike to a rather Gothic version of its earlier self.

As many other asylums Woodilee experienced a stark rise in numbers from the day of the first admission.[11] Built for 400 patients – 200 male, 200 female – the institution soon ran into a shortage of space. At the turn of the century the number of inmates already reached 750 men and women, not including the boarded out patients living in families or on farms all over Scotland. In 1907 there were over 500 beds for each sex, soon after the number rose to 1,150 in total. Woodilee catered for more patients only during the First World War, when due to the requisition of several Scottish asylums for war casualties 1,250 patients had to live on the premises.

with those formerly considered necessary adjuncts." Barony Parochial Lunatic Asylum Woodilee. Annual Report 1879, GCA GC 362.210941435 GLA, o. O., o. J., S. 8.

10 Regarding "Moral Treatment" see Digby (1983, 1985a, 1985b). For a very critical appraisal see Scull (1981).

11 There was a highly controversial discussion about the 'rise in lunacy' in Great Britain. The Scottish Lunacy Commissioners were critical of medical explanations – heredity and genetic degeneration – and favoured statistical explanations on the one hand and accounted better medical care in asylums for the rise in numbers on the other. A detailed report was published in one of the annual reports. See General Board of Commissioners in Lunacy for Scotland (1895) and Sibbald (1895).

Attendants and nurses

Everyday life in the asylum was structured and organized by nursing staff. According to meticulous schedules the daily face-to-face routines were executed by nurses and attendants as well as by non-medical staff.[12] This is probably true for large scale lunatic asylums at the turn of the 19th century in Western Europe and North America, as academic research has pointed out in detail in the last two decades. And this is definitely the case for Woodilee Asylum during the period 1875–1925. Although the physicians, and especially the physician superintendent, did set the gross guidelines[13], examined the patients and ordered therapies, the relation between patients and doctors was perfunctory at best[14]. Michel Foucault already pointed to the very unfavourable ratios of doctors to patients in his lectures on "psychiatric power".[15] Within the Scottish poor law asylums it was slightly better throughout the 19th century, but not to a large extent. In Woodilee, the ratio of doctors to patients was about 200–300 to 1, depending on the period under review. For a short time after the first admissions, the first superintendent had to care for about 400 patients, as he was the only physician on the premises. But except for the duration of the First World War, the ratio was never worse than 300 to 1 after the first few years. The gross numbers show, that there was scarce opportunity for close relationships between physicians and patients.[16] Having said that, the main workload with the patients lay on attendants and nurses The ratios of patients to nurses was 10–13 to 1 throughout the period. During the nearly fifty years I researched, the institution grew in size considerably and the staff numbers rose accordingly. In day-time the staff-patient ratio oscillated between 1 to 10 and 1 to 12. During nights, the ratio dropped. At the opening of

12 For this paper non-medical staff will not be considered in detail. Nevertheless it is important to remember that these cooks, maidens, artisans and craftsmen instructed the patients on many allotted tasks. The asylum in Woodilee maintained workshops as upholstery, a carpenter's workshop, a bootmaking shop, tailor's shop, farms, bakery and others, all of which were guided by non-medical staff.

13 These guidelines had to be in accordance with general recommended standard procedures issued by the General Board of Commissioners in Lunacy in Scotland. The parish printed several of these "general rules" for the asylum in Woodilee. See for example Glasgow District Asylum, Woodilee Lenzie (1900), in which a detailed workday's schedule and the hours to be observed in different workshops are printed.

14 Throughout the asylums the contact between physicians and patients was closer or more casual, depending on the wards in which the patients were placed as well as to their behaviour. But even in wards for restless and aggressive patients the doctor-patient-ratio did not allow much close contact. See for example the case of T. C., Margaret, NHSGGCA, HB-30-5-51, 17.

15 Foucault cites Leuret, who calculated that the "normal" head doctor had about 37 minutes per patient per year, while in some larger hospitals in France this decreased to a "maximum of eighteen minutes a year to each patient." Foucault (2006), p. 179–180.

16 Although in some cases the physicians and even the physician superintendent seemed to have put effort and time into relationships with patients and their relatives. See Gründler (2013), p. 246–260.

the institution in 1875, only two of the attendants were officially labeled "night attendants". But as a general rule, all female nurses and most of the male attendants had to sleep in the asylum during nights. Therefore in cases of emergency several personnel could be called up. Only during the First World War, with many male attendants and physicians on military duty and rising patient numbers, the ratios worsened drastically.[17]

Obviously, the nurses and attendants organized and supervised daily routines. They went out with the inmates to work in the fields. And they did put the patients to other "good use": cleansing, cooking and needlework. They guided the meals, the washing and most of the routine therapies. They were never "officially" in charge of the patients, but in everyday life they were.

Despite their importance, nurses and attendants were in the least favourable position inside the asylum system. They were sandwiched between a rock and a hard place. They had to follow the orders of the medical superintendent and other physicians and execute these orders on the patients. But while the doctors were so few and far away, the nursing staff had to take the physical and psychological backlash of those orders. They were the "first responders" and therefore more often the victims of physical outbursts and attacks than their doctoral counterparts.

This contributed a lot to the fact, that work in the asylum was considered as challenging, to say the least. It was difficult for superintendents to find men and women willing to take the job by heart. And it was even more difficult find personnel that was willing to keep it. During the period the physician superintendents complained about the constant flux of employees to the poor law bodies and committees. A few reasons can at least partly explain the problem. Certainly, one explanation is the bad payment. In the late 1870s it was reported:

> The scale of remuneration for ordinary attendants and nurses which has been adopted, and for which the Medical Superintendent would respectfully request the formal sanction of the Committee is, – for attendants from £28 to £40 per annum, and for nurses, from £14 to £20, according to experience and ability.[18]

In the 1880s and 1890s, male attendants started at about £30 per annum, while females got about £18.[19] And in 1910 salaries had not changed perceptibly.[20] Men still started at £30 per annum, women got even less pay with about £16 – depending on experience, the income could rise to £50, or £30

---

17   Research concerning other mental hospitals during the First World War show that downsizing the staff had serious consequences for daily life. In connection with food deprivation and overcrowding due to military requisition of asylums it was a factor in the rising mortality in some asylums during the war. See i. e. Crammer (1992) or Cherry (2003).

18   See Report of Medical Superintendent of Woodilee Asylum, 11.4.1876. In: Barony Parochial Board: Minutes of the BPB and Committees from 26th January 1876 to 28th December 1877, Vol. 3 [printed], GCA, D-Hew-2-2, 1A.

19   See for example Minutes of the Barony Parish Board and Committees from 28th December 1880 to 26th December 1881, Vol. 6 [printed], GCA, D-HEW-2-2, 5.

20   Pryor (1993) also points to the stagnant pay in mental health care around 1900. See also Brimblecombe (2005).

respectively.[21] Board and lodging was included in payment, but this rather worsened the situation. Lodging on the grounds was compulsory both for women for most men.[22] In the staff's perspective this meant, they were not much better positioned than the inmates in several perspective. First, it implied living in constant contact with and under close scrutiny of the medical superintendent. In the early years each leave had to be applied for, during the whole time these had to be documented in a register. And only in the 1890s nurses' homes were erected. Until then, nurses and attendants had to live in the asylum buildings itself, adjacent to the wards. The non-attractiveness of working in Woodilee was no surprise then. Particularly if one considers, that the opportunities of Glasgow – in terms of better paid jobs, self-determined life and amusement – lurked in plain sight. Therefore, the workforce in the asylum consisted mostly in the so called "lower orders" of society.[23] At least, the medical superintendents thought so. When James Rutherford applied for a new scale of remuneration for ordinary attendants and nurses in 1876 he underlined his request with the following remarks, in which he recapitulates the aforesaid and points to another explanation for high staff turnovers: "In connection with severe everyday restrictions [...] and the geographical location on the north-western outskirts of Glasgow and the special exigencies of the job, working as an asylum attendant or nurse was especially non attractive."[24] Rutherford realized how difficult life was for attendants and nurses, being forced to live in the asylum with little spare time, especially being so close to Glasgow. But he also pointed to a more fundamental problem of working in an asylum.

The job demanded a lot from employees. Since late 18th and early 19th century the institutions changed from custodial to curative institutions, stipulating new competences and skills as well as a different work understanding

---

21   But despite women earning about 50% to one-third less than their male counterparts, around 1900 the number of male attendants decreased significantly and caring for lunatics became female in Woodilee. This reflects an overall trend that care for the ill became feminized during the late 19th century. While in hospitals for the bodily ill this development began earlier and was implemented straightforward and more comprehensive, male attendants were replaced to a lesser extent in mental hospitals and remained an irreplaceable part of the workforce, although to a much lesser extent. See i.e. Schultheiss (2001); O'Lynn/Tranbarger (2007); O'Lynn (2007); Hawkins (2010).

22   Of course, this did not apply to non-medical staff like carpenters, the baker and the bootmaker.

23   This was in stark contrast to the requirements medical officers expected. Nurses and attendants were asked to be constant examples for good behaviour, friendliness and consideration for patients, as handbooks and instructions explained in detail. See Glasgow District Asylum, Woodilee Lenzie (1900) or Campbell Clark; McIvor Campbell; Turnbull; Urquhart (1885).

24   See Report of Medical Superintendent of Woodilee Asylum, 11.4.1876. In: Barony Parochial Board: Minutes of the BPB and Committees from 26th January 1876 to 28th December 1877, Vol. 3 [printed], GCA, D-Hew-2-2, 1A.

and ethos of nurses and attendants.[25] The special exigencies Rutherford alluded to were described in the "Red Handbook" for nurses and attendants.[26] And without going into too much detail, the requirements to men and women caring for lunatics in asylums were quite unrealistic. They should have been examples in every respect of human behaviour, always being patient, never loosing their temper. Retaliation, abusive language, mishandling or neglect were reasons for instant dismissal.[27] Despite the strenuous job description, these kinds of dismissals were rare in Woodilee. Instead, breaches of discipline lead to more staff being set free.[28] But rather than being dismissed, most members of staff resigned their positions in Woodilee on free will. During the first years of existence, nearly no months passed without several changes in staff. In some months up to 30% of the employees left Woodilee and took up work elsewhere.[29] The situation began to change in the 1890s, when measures to professionalize nursing were adopted. Courses for nurses and attendants, designed by the Medico-Psychological Association, were offered to interested members of staff. The courses were finished by an exam that officially certified successful candidates as mental nurses. The result of the certification remained ambiguous. Although the physicians got better-qualified staff, it allowed nurses and attendants to change positions within the realm of psychiatric care more easily, not least because it expanded during the whole period.

And another major factor for women leaving employment in an asylum was not even touched by professionalization or rising payments. Female nurses were strictly prohibited from marrying. This was of major significance for the continuing flux of staff. Being on the lower end of the social strata regarding

---

25 In many respects this account is simplistic. The change from custodial to curative was neither clear cut nor drastic. Many patients did not experience much change in therapies. And many old narratives of the treatment of lunatics before the advent of the Lunacy Laws seem to be rather founding myths of the psychiatric profession. An overview of the changes can be found for example Michael (2003); Scull (1993); Walton (1981). Nevertheless the changes in the legal, institutional and therapeutical setup in mid-Nineteenth century had intense consequences for nurses and attendants.

26 Campbell Clark; McIvor Campbell; Turnbull; Urquhart (1885). An earlier example, which pointed in the same direction, but being less detailed and tailored to the needs of administrative bodies, was Forbes Winslow (1877).

27 See Campbell Clark; McIvor Campbell; Turnbull; Urquhart (1885), p. 53–54 and 57–58. Also Forbes Winslow (1877), p. 5–8.

28 Thomas Gibson and William Meldrum were dismissed for harsh treatment of patients in April and May 1881 respectively. But during the period 1875 to 1921 there were only a few dozen dismissals for those reasons. Instead, more staff was dismissed for bad discipline and carelessness. See. Report Medical Superintendent, 19.4.1881 and 17.5.1881, in: Minutes of the Barony Parish Board and Committees from 28th December 1880 to 26th December 1881, Vol. 6 [printed], GCA, D-HEW-2-2, 5; Report Medical Superintendent, 20.12.1881, in: Minutes of the Barony Parish Board and Committees from 28th December 1880 to 26th December 1881, Vol. 6 [printed], GCA, D-HEW-2-2, 5; Report Medical Superintendent, 12.1.1880, in: Minutes of the Barony Parish Board and Committees from 30th December 1879 to 30th November 1880, Vol. 6 [printed], GCA, D-HEW-2-2, 4.

29 And more often than not they changed into industrial jobs.

payment and education, loosing employment because of marriage was a staggering perspective. At the turn of the century, many families in Glasgow still lived on economies of makeshift, in which each able member of the family had to contribute to the family's income.[30] Therefore, the nurses had to change employment at the latest when they decided to marry.[31] But more often they changed into jobs they could keep after marriage even before family life became a genuine option. As a return was barred, even if the child bearing and rearing period was over, and married nurses were not allowed to work in asylums a career as a nurse seemed even more disappointing and bleak.[32]

These remarks suggest, that conflicts due to bad payment, bad professional education and stress were implemented in the inner fabric of the asylum. A close reading of the case files should underline the conflictive nature of everyday life in asylums accordingly.

Relations between nurses and patients – the narratives in the case files

Case files in poor law asylums – and probably in other asylums as well – had a special purpose. On the one hand they were designed to broaden and extend medical knowledge and the understanding of mental illness. At the same time they served to describe and evaluate the development of individual patients. But on the other hand, as Peter Bartlett and others have convincingly argued, they also served administrative purposes.[33] In view of the information noted in the files it seems, that the design was more appropriate to the needs of the administration and statistics as for medical ones. For the administration, the case files played an important role in financial perspectives. With recourse to the files the local authorities could reclaim part of the cost of the care from national funds and demand refunds from other local poor law administrations. But more importantly, the case files had legal significance. They were written proof, that the patients were rightfully admitted to the asylum and kept there. They documented the need for therapy and institutionalization and they allowed national and local boards of control to check on the rightfulness. Accordingly, the General Commissioners in Lunacy for Scotland biannually checked each institution for the care of lunatics whether or not the files were correctly maintained and if the confinement of the patients was accurate. Due to this nature and purpose of the medical case files, the written narrative

---

30 A good starting point to economies of makeshift is King/Tomkins (2003). My own research on pauper lunatics emphasizers the importance of combining incomes within families as survival strategy well into the 20th century. See Gründler (2013).

31 Professionalizing made it easier for the nurses to change into private households or other forms of paid care service. Certificates were valid proof of good service and required knowledge.

32 The strict prohibition of marriage for female nurses and the enforced living on the grounds of the asylum was only relieved after the First World War.

33 See Bartlett (1999a; 1999b).

of relations between staff and patients consists mainly of tales of conflict and
distrust.

> When caught she deliberately knocked nurse Cartwright's spectacles out of her hand
> smashing them. [...] [S]he created a great disturbance in the large dining hall at tea-time,
> smashing several dishes, including a plate which she threw at nurse McKechnie, nar-
> rowly missing her [...]. She struggled violently when restrained + called the nurses mur-
> derers etc.[34]

The offensive woman in this case was named Margaret T.C. She spent about
14 months in Woodilee. In her medical certificate the doctors described her as
"dull and depressed" and "delusional in her ideas". She tried to commit suicide two years prior to her admission and was treated in Woodilee for five
weeks at that time. On admission the physician noted that she was "depressed,
nervous and apprehensive" and that she avoided conversation. During the 14
months, the doctor(s) in charge made twenty notes in her file. The first entries
characterized her mental state. On July, 16th 1921, eight weeks after admission, the physician notes: "this patient is truculent and secretive, and a source
of considerable anxiety to the nurses. She has been put on a red ticket since
admission [...]."[35] The "red ticket" signified her to be suicidal and therefore
under close watch by the nurses. The nurses informed the doctor in charge of
the worries the patient caused, and apparently he deemed the information
reliable enough to put it on record. After being transferred to the main building in August no changes occurred until early December. When she was informed of an internal transfer to the "observation dormitory" she "decamped"
but was quickly apprehended. A physical altercation evolved during this ap-
prehension and between the seventh and 14th December several attacks on
nurses, doctors and other patients arose. For furthers five months she at least
attacked staff and other inmates five times physically or verbally. In each of
these occurrences, nurses played a significant role, mainly perceived as victims[36] in the notes[37].

Having taken a female patient as example is not founded on a significantly more violent female population of the asylum. Violent outbursts and
attacks as well as verbal abuse and threatening were evenly distributed between male and female patients in Woodilee. While more men were described
as violent, abusive or threatening in behaviour in their respective medical
certificates, in everyday life within the compound of the asylum male and fe-

---

34   Note of 16.12.1921 in Case File T.C., Margaret, NHSGGCA, HB-30-5-51, 17.
35   Note of 16.7.1921 in Ibid.
36   But of course, there were stories that flipped the coin, especially in the bourgeois press.
     Those stories described the nurses and attendants as soulless and brutal, violent and
     overtaxed. But these narrations have to be analysed elsewhere.
37   The case notes of Margaret T.C. evoke many questions that cannot be addressed here.
     Foremost, within the notes there is a perceptible tension between the doctor's assessment
     of the patient, the nurses' narrations and the patient's perspective. Furthermore, there are
     clear indications that the narrowness and missing privacy in an asylum could change the
     behaviour of patients dramatically. And the case file gives ample evidence of the fact, that
     the physicians' supervision was perfunctory at best.

male patients behaved similarly. Margaret T. C. has been taken as an example for another reason. Her behaviour was archetypical in some respect. She, as many other inmates, had several short episodes of violent outbursts rather than being continuously violent or increasingly aggressive against members of staff. Furthermore, the days of non-violent behaviour outnumbered the violent ones by far. And lastly, Margaret T. C.'s attacks on staff and other patients were not severe or outrageous. Rather, the case notes hint at the instance that most of her outbursts were "provoked" or reactions to events that offended her. The doctor in charge informs the reader that she fled when she was informed of her transfer, had an outburst when she was reprimanded for eating food for other patients or should return a brush. However, this kind of quarrels and skirmishes certainly formed a picture of asylums as places of unruly behaviour and conflict.

Other examples underline the "real" danger for staff in asylums, an image that imprinted itself in the opinions of many contemporaries. One of these rare nevertheless lasting examples is that of James Y., a young man of 20 years.[38] He was admitted as a 15-year-old teenager in May 1915. His stay in Woodilee was characterized by a continuously rising curve of aggression and violence. During his five year long career he attacked several members of the staff and visitors physically. In 1917 he injured a member of the non-medical staff by throwing stones "without apparent reason". In 1918 he severely injured a young mother visiting the asylum. The following year he attacked his mother and sister "savagely" and in June 1920 he lashed out at a kitchen maid with a sweeping brush. In August of the same year, he attempted to murder the wife of one of the non-medical employees during a cricket game. Following this last escalation he was transferred to the Criminal Lunatic Department in Perth. Although he never seemed to have attacked nurses or attendants, occurrences of this kind must have had a profound impact on the medical staff. But one can assume, that it was not a lasting one. Cases as James Y. were swiftly dealt with in "normal" asylums. In Scotland, as well as England and Wales, a special department for homicidal lunatics was established following the Lunacy Act of 1857. Accordingly, patients who turned out to be extremely dangerous for others were transferred to Broadmoor in Berkshire or Perth in Scotland.

Margaret's and James' cases are two of many examples that could be quoted to demonstrate how relations unfold in the case files. They vividly manifest the physical and psychological violence nurses and attendants were exposed to. Mostly, the other files contain less graphic assaults and attacks – many of struggles to restrain patients in which both parties were hurt or other "accidental" occurrences. The stories told in the case files, then, are the rowdyish, garrulous, quarrelsome and violent ones. But there is another narration embodied in the silence of the sources. The purpose of the case files and the small amount of time to compile them makes the physicians concentrate on

38 For his case see letters concerning James Y., in: Letter Book, NHSGGCA, HB-30-7-24, pp. 270, 978, 986–987, 988.

the important events, on diagnoses, on the unexpected and the exceptional. As a consequence, the case files manifest more blanks, more omissions and more gaps than they produce information. The stories told in the case files are partial. The stories omitted in the files shed another spotlight on everyday life in asylums.

Resuming the case of Margaret T. C. underlines this point. Margaret stayed in Woodilee asylum for about 400 days. As presented before, during this time, the doctors recorded violent incidents on six days. Reading the case files the other way round, focussing on the blanks, this would imply, that on 394 days nothing worth recording happened. Perhaps this is a too euphemistic interpretation of the silence in the file. But the case files in Woodilee had the capacity to document any incidents involving physical altercations for legal consideration and for inspection. As mentioned before, a close network of control agencies for asylums existed in Scotland. A national body, the General Board of Commissioners in Lunacy for Scotland, had to inspect each asylum biannually. Furthermore, the local poor law administration had to establish committees that fortnightly met in Woodilee to inspect the books and decide on purchases and other matters. Moreover, members of these committees had to make inspections in the asylum once a week, taking patients' remonstrations and ensuring that everything was in order. Therefore it is safe to suggest, that Margaret did not attack or abuse nurses and attendants on said 394 days. Nearly all other case files point into the same direction. In not one of the 500 case files analysed for this paper one can find an indication for a patient that was permanently dangerous, abusive or violent. Rather, abuse and violence were episodic occurrences with the patients. Having said that, the case files only give hints on the nature of relations between nurses and attendants and patients. Mostly, the silence is the only thing we can use for interpretation. Again, the case of Margaret T. C. can serve as a typical example what happened in-between her violent episodes. For some time, she was under more or less constant supervision being on a red ticket due to her suicidal tendencies. Obviously Margaret resented the control being "truculent and resistive". But after a few weeks, she behaved much better and was working as a laundry maid. And she was transferred to the main building, where patients were housed that behaved "better". Apparently, she gained some trust in the nurses and kept peaceful.[39] However, although we do not know whether the relations between Margaret and her nurses were really friendly and cooperative or not, we at least know that they were nonviolent. In some other case files, the co-operation between staff and patients is explicitly depicted. Sarah B. B. was, although "abusive and threatening" after admission, continually "usefully employed" and "usually benevolent + good natured".[40] The same is true for

---

39   To one, she confided her emotions and feelings: "She expresses delusions of suspicion and persecution to the nurse." In this particular instance, the nurse figured as a trustworthy companion, an ally.
40   Case File Sarah B. B., NHSGGCA, HB-30-5-51, 16.

Richard B., who was treated for more than a year in Woodilee.[41] Even Agnes D., a 41 year old reeler, who was characterized as "one of the most troublesome patients in the house" behaved mostly well.[42] There were months-long periods, in which no outbursts were recorded and she was quite and amenable. One of the later entries of her treatment in Woodilee described her as "towards the nurses she is usually pleasant and fairly obliging". It is obvious, especially from Agnes D.'s case file, that the silence and the blanks are periods, in which the patients behaved more or less peaceful and well. But, of course, the case files still document the "official" perspective. The question remains, whether patients had different opinions and views on the relationship to nurses and attendants.

Relations between nurses and patients – the patients' perspectives

First of all, it is difficult ascertain the patient's view about nurses and attendants. As the case files themselves, the letters and notes written by patients, that were kept in the files, had a special purpose. The letters and notes, sometimes even drawings, were collected for two reasons. First, the physicians would use them to establish or differentiate their assessment. Letters to Queen and noblemen, surreal drawings or scribbled notes gave an insight to the muddled and disturbed minds of the patients. And secondly, these ego-documents were archived in the case files to emphasize to any inspector, committee member, supervisor or Commissioner in Lunacy the rightfulness of treatment and confinement in the asylum. Accordingly, one would expect that more letters with narratives of conflict survived as sources.

It is striking, that not many ego-documents of patients exist in the files at all. In the five hundred I looked into only about 40 contained actual letters or notes. It is unclear why there are so few. One of the reasons might be, that as a rule letters had to be sent to the addressee. Another conceivable cause is that after release or death of a patient, the administration returned all personal belongings to the nearest relatives. Having said that, it is also reasonable to suppose that either the physicians deemed the keeping unnecessary or that many ego-documents got lost while being kept.[43] However, the number of documents that originated from patients hands in the case files are little although from other archival sources it is obvious that patients were writing a lot.[44] The letters and notes that are still in the files rarely touch the relation-

---

41   Case File Richard B., NHSGGCA, HB-30–4–29, 11.
42   Case File Agnes D., NHSGGCA, HB-30-5-7, 43.
43   The case files were kept in an asylum building until the late 1980s when the institution closed. Only then the files were put into an archive.
44   Repeatedly the case files talk about the patients writing letters and notes to relatives and friends frequently, even to the queen or politicians. But even these latter letters did not survive in the files. The physicians' letter books describe some patients as frequent writers also, without one of the original letters surviving in the files.

ship with staff at all. The ones that do were mostly written by male patients, basically containing more or less serious complaints about staff behaviour.

One telling and explicit example is the letter Hugh sent to the General Commissioners in Lunacy for Scotland to remonstrate his treatment in Woodilee.[45] He was admitted two years prior to his complaint in 1917, behaved very well and worked with different groups, mostly indoors, according to his file. In his letter he elaborates that he stopped working. He then felt bullied by medical and nursing staff, which reduced his food and not getting his rations of tobacco. He picked out one attendant in his complaint:

> The attendant, called Mr. Smart, saw me smoking my pipe one day he was round here, and he said to me who gave you the tobacco for your pipe. I said some good friend that I have been good to myself. Well, he said to me if I know the ones that give you the tobacco, I will stop their tobacco. I never said anything, they have never gave me my tobacco back yet since I stop the work two months ago after me working hard for two long years polishing floors, making beds, scrubbing dining halls and polishing dancing halls and this is the treatment I am getting now.[46]

In the same letter he complained about a physician as well, but the attendants were his focus. He also remonstranced about the head attendant's behaviour who he accused of being violent against him, kicking him. The attendants in this instance appeared to be a natural enemy to the patient. Mr Smart tried to keep up discipline and order. As in the case files, in the letters kept by the institution the narrative focus was put on the conflicting side of the relations. One Robert C. reported in a letter written after his getaway: "[…] when I was admitted to Eastern District Hospital that night I got assaulted by a Male Attendant and was called a Bastard […]".[47] It is unclear what, if anything, happened in the matter. No letters of the medical staff are in the file. As Robert wrote to other poor law authorities as well, at least a formal investigation should have been made. As it was mandated legally that appeals as this one had to be reviewed and documented by the Commissioners of the General Board of Control for Scotland.[48] Of course, the truthfulness of Robert's claims cannot not be ascertained by reading the file.[49] Similarly to the case files then, the documents left by the patients and kept in the hospital archives tell us

45 Case File Hugh H., NHSGGCA, HB-30-4-42, p. 33.

46 Letter of 18.8.1917 in Case File Hugh H., NHSGGCA, HB-30-4-42, p. 33.

47 The patient was asking about the valuables he left behind when escaping and furthermore he demanded a compensation for his time in Woodilee. He deemed himself perfectly sane and his admission an injustice. Letter of 21.2.1932 in Case File Robert C., NHSGGCA, HB-30-4-51, 2.

48 The General Board of Control for Scotland was the legal successor of the General Board of Commissioners in Lunacy for Scotland from 1914 onwards.

49 That attendants could be the focus of imaginary accusations as well gets obvious in one last example. In a letter to a nurse one patient reported: "While in Duke St. Hospital […] I was thrown to the mercy of four attendants, beaten black, blue + bleeding, knocked + kicked about the bed + the floor, nearly throttled with locked mufflers, placed in a straight jacket + left all night in it. This occurred twice."12 As this was written in the context of various accusations against the nurse and a conspiracy theory one could easily understand why the doctors did not act upon his story. Still, that the patient used attend-

narratives of conflict. Patients and staff appear as antagonists, opponents in an adverse setting. But of course this is not only due to a certain medical or administrative directive only to keep notes and letters proving mental illness or the dangerousness of a patient. Both examples show, that the patients wrote about the conflicts – in both cases probably to underline their own agendas. Hugh H. wanted to be released and Robert C. wanted to be refunded for his work in Woodilee during his treatment. Therefore, narrating the conflicts with attendants and nurses were considered a useful means of achieving their respective goals.

And again, the gaps and the silence tell a different story. Robert and Hugh give only little evidence of conflict with staff. And Hugh in particular argues that he behaved well for two years, having no quarrels with staff, being polite and cooperative. And he implicitly underlines that most patients did get on well with the staff. Furthermore, there are no reports of clashes or arguments with staff in both of the patients' files. Robert was polite and cooperative as well during his time in Woodilee.[50] Obviously, there was no reason to write a complaint about good relationships between patients and staff. And even if letters existed that described the good and calm life in the asylum. What should have been the reason to keep them in the files?

Conclusion

As I have tried to show, there are two narratives about daily life in the asylum to be found in patients' case files. On the one hand, they tell a tale of two conflicting parties. Nursing staff versus patients. In the case files the doctors mostly did put the blame on patients illnesses. As statistics show, attendants or nurses were made responsible for arguments and skirmishes very rarely. The files seem to document that life in the asylum was violent, rowdyish, full of dispute and conflict. On the other hand, the silence of many files on clashes and unruly behaviour and the seldom mentioning of serious fighting tell another tale of life in the asylum without words: one of order, peace and calm. Of course, one cannot be sure how much the physician kept quiet about. But it seems reasonable to assume, that most incidents were noted.

A very similar narrative is told by patients' ego-documents. In complaints and letters attendants often constituted the adversaries of patients. Two points that I could not discuss in detail stand out: Firstly, males made all complaints. Secondly, no female nurses were targets of complaints. Whether this was due

---

ants to tell his story implicates he experienced a rather tense relation to the nursing staff in Woodilee.

50 Jessie B. H., the daughter of a minister and a nurse herself, wrote the only letter of a female patient touching on the topic. Her tone was rather subservient, she begged the medical superintendent to allow visits by her family. Whether this gender difference was normal inside Woodilee remains unclear, because I found only her letter. But the difference would be in accordance with wider societal gender stereotype and behaviour in Victorian Britain.

to gender norms, male self-perception or archival accidents remains unclear until further research is done. Anyway, the written story in the ego-documents is one of conflict. But again, the silence is interesting. Even in the examples I presented, life before and after the complaints seemed to have been calm and cooperative.

Therefore, as on the outdoors, conflict and cooperation co-existed in Woodilee, with the normal mode of life being cooperation. It is a story that can be found in official reports of the General Commissioners in Lunacy for Scotland, of the medical staff or the poor law authorities as well. As no diaries or ego documents of the nursing staff exist, there is no way to check whether attendants and nurses experienced life in Woodilee in a similar or different way and how these experiences changed. However, the two narratives of conflict and cooperation exist simultaneously in all archival resources of this asylum. This concurrence cannot be dissipated. Life in the institution was complex and changing, and this ambiguity should rather be embraced than dissipated in a futile attempt.

Bibliography

Archival sources

Glasgow City Archives (GCA)

Barony Parochial Board/Council (D-Hew)
Parish of Glasgow Council (D-Hew)

NHS Greater Glasgow and Clyde Archives (NHSGGCA)

Barony Pauper Lunatic Asylum, Woodilee (HB-30)

Printed sources

Campbell Clark, Alexander; McIvor Campbell, Charles; Turnbull, A.R.; Urquhart, A.R.: Handbook for the Instruction of Attendants on the Insane. Prepared by a Sub-Committee of the Medico-Psychological Association Appointed at a Branch Meeting Held in Glasgow on the 21st February 1884. London 1885.
Forbes Winslow, Lyttleton S.: Handbook for the Attendants of the Insane. London 1877.
Glasgow District Asylum, Woodilee Lenzie: General Management of the Asylum, and General Rules for the Guidance of Attendants. Glasgow 1900.
John Sibbald: Memorandum for the General Board of Lunacy for Scotland, On the Increase in the Number of the Insane on the Register of the General Board of Lunacy for Scotland, with special reference to the Allegation that it indicates an Increased Prevalence of Insanity, in: Alleged Increasing Prevalence of Insanity in Scotland. Supplement to the Thirty-Sixth Annual Report of the General Board of Commissioners in Lunacy for Scotland. Edinburgh 1895, p. 16–56.

General Board of Commissioners in Lunacy: Supplement to Thirty-sixth Annual Report, on Alleged Increasing Prevalence of Insanity in Scotland. Edinburgh 1895.

Secondary research literature

Bartlett, Peter: The Poor Law of Lunacy. The Administration of Pauper Lunatics in Mid-Nineteenth-Century England. London; Washington 1999a.

Bartlett, Peter: The Asylum and the Poor Law: The Productive Alliance. In: Melling, Joseph; Forsythe, Bill (ed.): Insanity, Institutions, and Society, 1800–1914: A Social History of Madness in Comparative Perspective. London; New York 1999b, p. 48–67.

Beveridge, Allan: Life in the Asylum. Patient's Letter from Morningside, 1873–1908. In: History of Psychiatry 9 (1998), S. 431–469.

Beveridge, Allan; Williams, Morag: Inside "The Lunatic Manufacturing Company". The Persecuted World of John Gilmour. In: History of Psychiatry 13 (2002), 49, p. 19–49.

Braunschweig, Sabine: Einleitung. In: Braunschweig, Sabine (ed.): Pflege – Räume, Macht und Alltag. Beiträge zur Geschichte der Pflege. Zürich 2006a, p. 9–13.

Braunschweig, Sabine (ed.): Pflege – Räume, Macht und Alltag. Beiträge zur Geschichte der Pflege. Zürich 2006b.

Braunschweig, Sabine: Sexuelle Zwischenfälle – ein Störfaktor im psychiatrischen Pflegealltag der ersten Hälfte des 20. Jahrhunderts? In: Hähner-Rombach, Sylvelyn (ed.): Alltag in der Krankenpflege. Geschichte und Gegenwart / Everyday Nursing Life, Past and Present. Stuttgart 2009, p. 147–167.

Brimblecombe, Neil: Asylum nursing in the UK at the end of the Victorian era: Hill End Asylum. In: Journal of Psychiatric and Mental Health Nursing 12 (2005), p. 57–63.

Brimblecombe, Neil: Asylum nursing as a career in the United Kingdom, 1890–1910. In: Journal of Advanced Nursing 55 (2006), p. 770–777.

Cherry, Steven: Mental Health Care in Modern England: The Norfolk Lunatic Asylum / St. Andrew's Hospital C. 1810–1998. Bury St. Edmunds, Suffolk 2003.

Christians, Annemone; Kramer, Nicole: Who Cares? Eine Zwischenbilanz der Pflegegeschichte in zeithistorischer Perspektive. In: Archiv für Sozialgeschichte 54 (2014), p. 395–415.

Crammer, John: Extraordinary Deaths of Asylum Inpatients During the 1914–1918 War. In: Medical History 36 (1992), p. 430–41.

D'Antonio, Patricia: Revisiting and Rethinking the Rewriting of Nursing History. In: Bulletin of the History of Medicine 73 (1999), p. 268–290.

D'Antonio, Patricia; Fairman, Julie A.; Whelan, Jean C. (ed.): Introduction. In: D'Antonio, Patricia; Fairman, Julie A.; Whelan, Jean C. (ed.): Routledge Handbook of the History of Nursing. Abingdon; New York 2013, p. 1–8.

Digby, Anne: Changes in the Asylum. The Case of York, 1777–1815. In: Economic History Review 36 (1983), p. 218–239.

Digby, Anne: Madness, Morality and Medicine. A Study of the York Retreat 1796–1914. Cambridge u. a. 1985a.

Digby, Anne: Moral Treatment at the Retreat, 1796–1846. In: Bynum, W. F.; Porter, Roy; Shepherd, Michael (ed.): The Anatomy of Madness. Essays in the History of Psychiatry. Institutions and Society. London; New York 1985b, p. 52–72.

Foucault, Michel: Psychiatric Power. Lectures at the Collège de France, 1973–1974. Edited by Jaques Lagrange. Basingstoke 2006.

Goffman, Erving: Asylums. Essays on the Social Situation of Mental Patients and Other Inmates. New York 1961.

Gründler, Jens: Armut und Wahnsinn. "Arme Irre" und ihre Familien im Spannungsfeld von Psychiatrie und Armenfürsorge in Glasgow, 1875–1921. München 2013.

Hähner-Rombach, Sylvelyn (ed.): Alltag in der Krankenpflege. Geschichte und Gegenwart / Everyday Nursing Life, Past and Present. Stuttgart 2009.

Hawkins, Sue: Nursing and Women's Labour in the Nineteenth Century: The Quest for Independence. Milton Park; New York 2010.

Hide, Louis: Gender and Class in the English Asylum, 1890–1914. Basingstoke 2014.

King, Steven; Tomkins, Alannah (ed.): The Poor in England 1700–1850: An Economy of Makeshifts. Manchester; New York 2003.

Ledebur, Sophie: Schreiben und Beschreiben. Zur epistemischen Funktion von psychiatrischen Krankenakten, ihrer Archivierung und deren Übersetzung in Fallgeschichten. In: Berichte zur Wissenschaftsgeschichte 34 (2011), p. 102–124.

Michael,Pamela: Care and Tretament of the Mentally Ill in North Wales 1800–200. Cardiff 2003.

Nolan, Peter, Reflections of a Mental Nurse in the 1950s. In: History of Nursing Society Journal 5 (1994–5), p. 3.

Nolan, Peter: A History of Mental Health Nursing. Cheltenham 1998.

Nolte, Karen: Gelebte Hysterie. Erfahrung, Eigensinn und psychiatrische Diskurse im Anstaltsalltag um 1900. Frankfurt/Main, new York 2003.

Nolte, Karen: Querulantenwahnsinn. "Eigensinn" oder "Irrsinn"? In: Fangerau, Heiner; Nolte, Karen (ed.): "Moderne" Anstaltspsychiatrie im 19. und 20. Jahrhundert. Legimation und Kritik. Stuttgart 2006, p. 395–410.

O'Lynn, Chad E.; Russell E. Tranbarger (ed.): Men in Nursing: History, Challenges, and Opportunities. New York 2007.

O'Lynn, Chad E.: History of Men in Nursing. A Review. In: O'Lynn, Chad E.; Russell E. Tranbarger (ed.): Men in Nursing: History, Challenges, and Opportunities. New York 2007, p. 5–42.

Pryor, E.H.: A Century of Caring. Forest Healthcare Trust. Suffolk 1993.

Reaume, Geoffrey: Accounts of Abuse of Patients at the Toronto Hospital for the Insane, 1883–1937. In: Canadian Bulletin of Medical History 14 (1997), 1, p. 65–106.

Reaume, Geoffrey: Remembrance of Patients Past. Patient Life at the Toronto Hospital for the Insane, 1870–1940. Toronto; Oxford 2000.

Schultheiss, Katrin: Bodies and Souls: Politics and the Professionalization of Nursing in France 1880–1922. Cambridge, Mass.; London 2001.

Scull, Andrew: Moral Treatment Reconsidered: Some Sociological Comments on an Episode in the History of British Psychiatry. In: Scull, Andrew: Madhouses, Mad-Doctors and Madmen. The Social History of Psychiatry in the Victorian Era. London 1981, p. 105–120.

Scull, Andrew: The Most Solitary of Afflictions. Madness and Society in Britain, 1700–1900. London 1993.

Smith, Leonard D.: "Levelled to the Same Common Standard?" Social Class in the Lunatic Asylum. In: Ashton, Owen; Fyson, Robert; Roberts, Stephen (ed.): The Duty of Discontent. Essays for Dorothy Thompson. London; New York 1995, p. 142–166.

Smith, Leonard D.: "Cure, Comfort and Safe Custody". Public Lunatic Asylums in Early Nineteenth Century. London; New York 1999.

Smith, Leonard D.: "Your Very Thankful Inmate". Discovering the Patients of an Early County Lunatic Asylum. In: Social History of Medicine 21 (2008), 2, p. 237–252.

Walton, John K.: The Treatment of Pauper Lunatics in Victorian England: The Case of Lancaster Asylum, 1816–1870. In: Scull, Andrew (ed.): Madhouses, Mad-Doctors and Madmen. The Social History of Pychiatry in the Victorian Era. London 1981, p. 166–200.

Children and Young People in the Post-War Period as Patients in Psychiatric Child Observation Units. The Example of Innsbruck

Sylvelyn Hähner-Rombach

Summary

This essay deals with one group of psychiatric patients of whom notice has scarcely been taken during the period after the Second World War. Using the example of the patient files of the Innsbruck child observation unit, I primarily intend to show how children and young people with behavioural difficulties became psychiatric patients and what time spent in this station meant for them. These are the results of a recently completed medical history research project, whose options for nursing history are sketched out in a research outlook.

Introduction

Paediatric psychiatry is one of the fields which, in the light of its National Socialist past, had to be reconstructed, so to speak, after the Second World War. A characteristic of its development after 1945 was that new professions pushed into this area or were needed by it. For example, one can consider psychologists or remedial teachers for the therapeutic and diagnostic activities and teachers or social workers for the actual active care. This means that paediatric psychiatry is at the intersection of medicine, (special) education and social work. The children and young people who visited these institutions were not only patients but also "cases" for social workers and special and remedial teachers. The following essay concentrates on how, after World War 2, children and young people became patients of a special psychiatric or remedial education institution and which consequences that stay could have for them. After a brief depiction of the state of research, the "child observation unit" will be presented and the development of paediatric psychiatric institutions sketched out. A description of the facilities in Innsbruck follows on from this and then the affected children are briefly introduced and the sample under investigation presented. This is followed by an evaluation of the referral diagnoses and the initiators of the referral to answer the question of how children became patients of an observation station. Questions pertaining to the function of an observation unit and factors influencing these functions follow this up. The investigation of the discharge locations offers a first look at the consequences of the stay for the children, which will be examined in a targeted manner. A research outlook completes the essay.

Research situation

Whilst there is a large range of new research papers on adult psychiatry in the German-speaking world, research into the history of paediatric psychiatry is still at a very early stage. Institutional paediatric psychiatry has primarily been investigated in the standard work by Castell et al.[1] However, this only deals with the period between 1937 and 1961. The thematic alignment of this work means that child observation units are not taken into account. In other works, they have only been approached in a very minor way.[2] The research situation is better for the inter-war period. In particular, the facilities at the Charité[3] in Berlin and at Tübingen University Hospital[4] have been researched in more detail. Patient files have also been included in the investigation. There are also regional studies available for Hesse[5] and Bavaria[6]. However, these also remain as much on the institutional level as those from Switzerland, for which smaller works are available for the Jurasüdfuss[7] and Zürich[8] regions. For the period after 1945, research in the German-speaking world shows even greater deficits. If one tries to find anything on paediatric psychiatric institutions, results usually come as part of the history of an institution, for example in the monograph on the Bremen clinic, whose paediatric department was taken into account more adequately than in many other descriptions.[9] Thus, one has to look for individual pieces of the puzzle in order to gain an overview of the development of in-patient paediatric psychiatric institutions. Of particular help are the contemporary periodicals[10], which contain occasional reports from individual institutions. With the exception of the named examples of

---

1   Castell (2003).
2   One example is the Wittenauer Heilstätten, see Beddies/Dörries (1999).
3   Kölch (2002).
4   Köhnlein (2001).
5   Keim (1999).
6   Rexroth (2011). The title makes it clear that historical treatment of this is very limited.
7   Schaffner-Hänny (1997).
8   Zürrer-Simmen (1994).
9   Engelbracht (2004).
10 The "Zeitschrift für Kinderforschung", which was first published in January 1896 under the name "Die Kinderfehler. Zeitschrift für Pädagogische Pathologie und Therapie in Haus, Schule und sozialem Leben", existed until 1944, when it was discontinued. It took twelve years, i.e. until 1956, for the "Jahrbuch für Jugendpsychiatrie und ihre Grenzgebiete" to appear as the successor to the "Zeitschrift für Kinderforschung". The "Jahrbuch" was issued a total of eight times between 1956 and 1971. The "Zeitschrift für Kinder- und Jugendpsychiatrie" then followed on. Since 1973, it has been published regularly under this name. The "Praxis der Kinderpsychologie und Kinderpsychiatrie. Zeitschrift für analytische Kinderpsychologie, Psychotherapie und Psychagogik in Praxis und Forschung" has been published since 1952. Finally, the Swiss "Zeitschrift für Kinderpsychiatrie – Acta Paedopsychiatrica" should be mentioned, which was founded in 1934, and was published until 1994 under the name "Acta paedopsychiatrica: europäische Zeitschrift für Neuropsychiatrie, Psychologie und Psychotherapie des Kindes- und Jugendalters".

Tübingen and Berlin, children and young people have, up to now, been of little interest to researchers in the history of psychiatry.

Child observation units

Firstly, the structure and tasks of such a unit should be sketched out.

What is a child observation unit?

The designation of a psychiatric or remedial education department or unit, in which children and young people stay for a varying period of time, was not standardised. As such, in the following essay, the term "child observation unit" will be used. A stay in such a station was primarily for observation, psychological testing and evaluation. In many cases, the children and young people also received therapy there. Their creation was considered progress and was welcomed warmly by the youth welfare offices.[11] This is because they offered the possibility or hope, which was not or rarely available previously, of "viewing" and "classifying" problematic children and young people by medical experts, in order to determine their future place of residence more adequately.

The stations were managed by psychiatrists or paediatricians. In Switzerland, in particular, they were run by remedial teachers. Additional personnel would have included psychologists, along with child psychotherapists at a later time. In the early period, nurses, child nursers and kindergarten teachers would have also been a part of the team. After the Second World War, large numbers of child care workers and remedial teachers were employed in the actual, everyday observation and occupation of the children, as well as nurses for night-time work. Almoners, who would be later termed social workers, are also mentioned. In most cases, for those children of school age, a school (i. e. the employment of teachers who worked in specially-created teaching rooms) with various educational levels was set up.

This wide range of different professions makes it clear that the child observation units were a more or less highly specialised area, depending on the facility. The number of people involved gives the impression that these units were very large, although the opposite is actually the case. In the period under investigation, the capacity was usually between four (with individual "nurse-

---

11 For example, in 1959, the Gustav Werner Stiftung zum Bruderhaus, a major diocesan care home provider in Württemberg, took the demand of its "institutional doctor", who had been employed since 1953, into account, and set up a small observation unit for children, for whom it was not clear for which home they were suitable. The employment of a doctor (and additional academic) and the creation of the observation unit can be considered an innovation when viewing the history of care homes. Cf. Hähner-Rombach (2013), pp. 85 f., 90 f.

ries") and around 52 (in Marburg an der Lahn) children, and, in exceptional cases, even more.[12] On average, a child observation unit had 20 to 25 beds.

Development of child psychiatric institutions in the German-speaking area

Until the beginning of the 20th century, many of the increasing number of psychiatric units lacked departments for accepting children. Those who were referred there were – to the great dismay of the psychiatrists – often housed with adults. They were usually female units, but, there too, situations could occur which were wholly unsuitable for children and young people. With only a few exceptions, it was not until the end of the 19th century that these young-sters were perceived as a separate group of patients, for whom there should be special facilities or at least spaces.

The very early foundations of institutions[13] and "departments" for chil-dren[14] were the first special facilities for mentally handicapped and/or epilep-

---

12   For example, in the Bonn unit, there is talk of 60 beds. Whether these were actually part of the observation unit are not is unknown. Cf. Orth (1989), p. 10.

13   The first "Hospital for feeble-minded and psychically abnormal children" was opened in Wildberg in Württemberg in 1853. Cf. Köhnlein (2001), p. 33 f. The sanatorium and mental hospital "Levana" in Baden near Vienna was founded in 1856, but only remained open until 1866. Cf. Kirmsse (1908), pp. 307–315. A child educational institution (termed the "Städtische Idiotenanstalt") was opened in Berlin in 1888 and was, for the period, an "innovative and progressive remedial education concept for the promotion and educa-tion of 'feeble-minded' and 'psychopathic' children to give them the greatest possible independence". Children "capable of education" were taught in five rising classes of the hospital's own remedial school. The „Idiotenanstalt" was renamed as the „Heil- und Er-zeihungsanstalt" in 1915. Beddies/Dörries (1999), p. 77. By 1923/1924, only the children "capable of education and development" were retained and thus, in 1925, the name was changed to the "Erziehungsanstalt der Wittenauer Heilstätten". Beddies/Dörries (1999), p. 78.
     In 1919, the Kinderheilanstalt Buch was set up with a "neurological department" with 63 beds for "mentally ill, psychopathic and feeble-minded" children. This became a part of the Wittenauer Heilstätten (educational home) in 1934. From this point on, besides chil-dren "capable of education", children "incapable of education" between seven and 16 years, along with "feeble-minded" children under seven years were referred to it. "The educational home placed these children together in an observation department, which was primarily used as a transit unit." From there, the children were sent to homes and institutions hospitals across Brandenburg. In 1938, the educational institution of the Wit-tenauer Heilstätten received "in addition to the existing remedial education department and the special school, its own neurological-psychiatric department and a polyclinic termed the 'field hospital'." In 1941, the section of the Wittenauer Heilstätten termed the "educational home including the paediatric nerve clinic" was separated off and contin-ued as an independent hospital, the "Städtische Nervenklinik für Kinder". Cf. Beddies/ Dörries (1999), p. 79f. The term "Wiesengrund" was an official part of the name in the 1950s. Cf. Beddies/Dörries (1999), p. 81.

14   The institution in Frankfurt am Main, founded in 1864 and frequently deemed to have been the first child psychiatric department, was, according to Castell, not a department, but the start of the efforts by the psychiatrist Heinrich Hoffmann to give children and

tic children and young people, as well as experiments and early attempts to meet the needs of these age groups somewhat better in the existing adult institutions. The first paediatric psychiatric instruction manual was published by the Freiburg psychiatrist Hermann Emminghaus in 1887.[15] This was followed in 1898 by the foundation of the periodical "Die Kinderfehler" which, still dominated by educationalists, offered a means of publication for the new so-called "child research".

Castell and others state that the first separate department for children and young people was the "Städtische Klinik für Geisteskranke in Frankfurt", founded in 1900 by the doctor Emil Sioli (1852–1922).[16] After the turn of the century, out-patient consultancy offices appeared in the major cities for children with "educational difficulties, developmental problems or psychological abnormalities".[17] During the same period, the first observation departments for young people, so-called care pupils, were set up, for example in Göttingen in 1907.[18]

During the period of the First World War, its effects and consequences on children and young people led to an increasing number of institutions for the observation, examination and treatment of children and young people perceived as troublesome by psychiatrists. The development of laws for the protection of young people in the inter-war years, legitimising access to care pupils, encouraged further foundations of institutions in the major cities. After the Second World War, the large numbers of displaced people and fleeing children and young people led to a possibly even more intense social perception of these groups, who, in the years the followed, were regarded as having the potential to be dangerous. These also included the many children born outside wedlock and children sired by occupying forces, who also seemed to threaten the make-up of society.

The setup of paediatric psychiatric institutions was also caused, on the one hand, by the course of time and, on the other, by the professionalisation attempts by paediatric psychiatrists. Firstly, they acquired new patient groups, i.e. children and young people, and "thus increased the influence of psychiatry and the psychiatrist in society".[19] In addition, they used the new patients for the training of the would-be paediatric psychiatrists. In so doing, they made use of the contemporary problems (overfull psychiatric hospitals, wars,

---

young people their own hospital, run by him. – Castell (2003), p. 404f. – Stutte characterised it as the oldest child psychiatry-oriented hospital department in Germany, cf. Stutte (1960), pp. 194–202.

15 Emminghaus (1887).

16 Castell (2003), p. 405. The foundation of the University of Frankfurt am Main in 1914 meant that, in 1919, this paediatric department was the first "Department for paediatric psychiatry at a German university." Castell (2003), p. 406. It was, according to Matron, "conceived as a clinical observation unit for all kinds of mentally ill or feeble-minded children." Matron (2012), p. 79.

17 Köhnlein (2001), p. 38 f.

18 Köhnlein (2001), p. 39.

19 Köhnlein(2001), p. 152.

post-war years) and made society aware of the necessity of maintaining order and security. In this area, they were certainly successful. This was, in turn, aided by the appropriate laws (Laws for the Well-Being of Young People – "Jugendwohlfahrtsgesetze") in the Weimar Republic and in the post-war years. Since that time, the paediatric psychiatrists have been able to maintain and expand their status as experts for a long period with more or less no opposition.

The specialities of the units diverged to a large extent, as could be seen as early as the early post-war years. Whilst, for example, the Bremen child observation unit, which was set up in 1949, had a liberal orientation appropriate to its American support[20], the Innsbruck unit is on record as having a "repressive-restorative (remedial) education policy" under the authoritarian leadership of Maria Nowak-Vogl.[21] The concurrence of completely different concepts pertaining to the handling and treatment of children and young people with behavioural difficulties was widespread and – putting German-speaking Switzerland carefully to one side for a moment – was more or less typical for the post-War years, and not just in this area. The alignment of the appropriate unit was very strongly dependent on the person running it. The generation of paediatric psychiatrists not socialised under the National Socialist regime generally had an easier task in being more open to simpler, alternative therapeutic concepts. The general delay experienced in exploring new paths in paediatric psychiatry (and in home care) was also connected to the fact that the "rediscovery" of the methods discussed and developed in the inter-war years required a certain period of time after 1945. Only the experiment in removing the appearance of a psychiatric clinic from the paediatric units to increase acceptance was taken up again very quickly after the way. However, this was the result of the professional interests of the medical directors of these units. This could also be the reason why the affiliation of a closed department to a paediatric psychiatric institution, such as in Marburg, was the exception rather than the rule. The intention of avoiding the creation of the impression of a psychiatric clinic department was implemented in Marburg by moving into a villa.

The Innsbruck child observation unit

Shortly after the end of the Second World War, a room was created for the observation of children in the Innsbruck psychiatric university hospital, from which a separate unit was created outside the hospital site in 1954. The psychiatrist and remedial teacher Maria Nowak-Vogl became the head of the unit. The purpose of the station was to give children with behavioural difficulties who had been under observation recommendations for further measures.

---

20   Cf. Engelbracht (2004), p. 134 ff.
21   Ralser (2013), p. 40.

As, apart from the complete set of patient files, there are barely any documents available relating to the unit, little is known about its actual development. In 1954, besides Nowak-Vogl, one child care worker worked full-time there, one part-time and there was also a teacher.[22] A patient file of 1953 talks of seven beds.[23] The moving out of the unit in 1954 saw an increase to 21 spaces, with two groups for boys and one for girls.[24] This meant that the Innsbruck institution was one of the larger child observation units of the early period.[25] A parenting advisory office and out-patients' unit[26] were connected to this, which, in some cases, were the first of call for worried parents and also advised hospitalisation of some of the children passing through. By 1958, a psychologist was also employed. The number of child care workers increased[27], and, before 1961, a second teacher was employed in the unit's own school, as two classes had been set up.[28] The unit remained independent until 1979, when it was incorporated back into the university hospital.

Maria Nowak-Vogl's unit was not only the only one in the Tyrol, but the only in the whole of western Austria. Its significance and standing in caregiving cannot be emphasised strongly enough. As Nowak-Vogl also taught at the Institute for Education of the University of Innsbruck and trained home care workers, as well as maintaining contacts to the educational homes in the region, her influence extended far beyond the unit.[29] During the discussions on abuse in homes during the post-War years, the Innsbruck child observation unit was also brought into the spotlight. Maria Nowak-Vogl was criticised to a great extent in this regard. Former patients said that they had been used there for trials of medicines. However, the text below does not deal with this aspect.

---

22 Cf. Vogl (1954).
23 TLA number 2300.
24 Cf. Vogl (1961), p. 38.
25 For example, the Psychiatrisch-Neurologischen Universitätsklinik in Vienna was expanded to 12 beds in 1953. Cf. Spiel (1977), p. 3.
26 Cf. Vogl (1954).
27 Thus, documents from 1961 mention three groups, stating that each group had its own care workers, meaning that the institution had at least three care workers. Cf. Vogl (1961), p. 38.
28 Cf. Vogl (1961), p. 38.
29 Cf. Ralser (2013), p. 28 f.

Make-up of the investigation sample and brief characterisation of the children and young people

Between 1949 and 1987, a a total of 3,606 children and young people stayed in the unit, of whom around 63 percent were boys and 37 percent girls.[30] From the complete documentation, ten percent of the files were chosen at random for the analysis[31], with a roughly even gender distribution[32]. This means that 362 files were evaluated. The following section presents part of this evaluation.

Of the boys, 13.7 percent visited the unit multiple times, whilst the amount of girls was lower – 9.6 percent. More than 60 percent of the children and young people taken in came from families with two parents, although some-times these were stepfathers and stepmothers. Foster parents came second (almost 18 percent), followed by single parents (almost 14 percent). The pro-portion of children born out of wedlock was around 17 percent. Of those, the youth welfare office was appointed guardian and was the primary influence on the lives of these children. In total, the families of the children and young people were more mixed socially than one might assume, i. e. there was no majority of lower-class families, whose children were treated in the unit. The average age of the boys and girls rose over the decades from 10.6 years in the 1950s to 13.4 years in the 1980s, although boys were often taken in at a younger age than girls. Most children were in the unit for between 57 and 112 days (40.9 percent), following by those who stayed for between 22 and 56 days (35.6 percent). In third place were the 12.7 percent who stayed between seven and 21 days. Over the four decades under investigation, the average length of stay increased from 42.2 days in the period between 1949 and 1959 to an av-erage of 74.3 days between 1980 and 1989. However, in the last decade, it was considerably shorter than the three preceding decades. The slower rise in the average length of stay in the last decade correlates to the fall in admissions, which is particularly noticeable in the last decade. If, in the period from 1949 to 1959, 108 children of the sample were admitted and even 122 between 1960 and 1969, the number of admissions between 1970 and 1979 fell to 84 and finally, in the period between 1980 and 1989, to 48 children. This means that, the further forward one goes in the period under investigation, the more therapeutic alternatives there were, but also that the stays become shorter,

30 All the observation units which provided data stated that there were considerably more male patients than female. For example, in 1953, 230 children were taken in to the obser-vation department of the clinic in Essen, of whom 76 were girls (33 percent) and 154 were boys (around 67 percent). Cf. Bleckmann (1956), p. 9. In 1961, 69 percent of the patients at the paediatric psychiatric department of the Psychiatrische und Neurolo-gische Klinik at Heidelberg University were boys and 31 percent were girls. Cf. Müller-Küppers (1962), p. 169.
31 Cf. Buchholz (2011), p. 278 ff.
32 In the sample under investigation, 62.4 percent were boys and 37.6 percent were girls.

even if, in the last decade, some extremely long stays of several months increased the average.[33]

Some children, particularly girls, had been the victims of sexual abuse for a considerable period before their admission. Many only had a rudimentary education, as the parents or foster parents did not ensure they attended school regularly or because the children played truant. Some of them had already experienced foster care several times before their admission, sometimes under the worst material conditions with regard to their clothing, nutrition or cleanliness. The children had also frequently experienced physical violence from parents or guardians. Some of them came to the unit from orphanages or children's homes as the problems with them made a further stay in the home apparently impossible. In other words: A considerable proportion of the children and young people had a past history when they arrived at the unit, which had a massive influence on them.

What led up to admission?

To answer the question of why children and young people were admitted to the unit, it is first necessary to look at the diagnoses of those involved. A second look shows that, behind the term "diagnosis", there was frequently a conglomerate of admission reasons, symptoms and diagnoses over the period under examination.

Reasons for admission

To aid clarity, the following section only quantifies and differentiates between those diagnoses and admission reasons which occurred more than 20 times. Table 1 shows the quantitative distribution of these named and assigned diagnoses and admission reasons in the sample between 1949 and 1989. It should be noted that these are frequently parts of multiple mentions, which were counted individually.

---

33 For information on the parameters influencing the routines of psychiatric examination of these children, cf. Hähner-Rombach [to be published in 2017].

Tab. 1: Quantitative distribution of diagnoses by frequency and gender in the period between 1949 and 1989

Diagnoses	Male	Female	Total
Group 1: Organic faults and impairments:	80	36	116
Of which oligophreniae	33	25	57
Of which epilepsy	19	5	24
Of which organic brain damage	28	7	35
Group 2: Educational problems	60	23	83
Group 3: Reactive problems	48	32	80
Of which enuresis/encopresis	40	21	61
Group 4: Anti-social behaviour incl. delinquency, neglect	44	28	72
Of which sexuality	3	12	15
Group 5: Psychopathic attributions	35	17	52
Neuroses, psychasthenia, personality issues	30	18	48
Puberty problems/defiance	19	18	37
School problems + underperformance issues	22	14	36
Social problems	20	14	34
Deprivation	19	9	28
Housing issue	16	8	24

Source: Own calculations

Organic problems and impairments (oligophreniae, epilepsy, brain damage) were the most common reasons for both sexes, with a total of 116 mentions. The second most common (83 mentions) were educational problems, which comprised both a lack of education by the parents/guardians and so-called "educational difficulties" of the children and young people. The frequency with which education problems were stated is surely also linked to the fact that the initiative for the admission of these children primarily came from parents.

In the case of so-called reactive problems, I counted the cases of enuresis and encopresis specially, as they occurred with such frequency and because their causes were interpreted differently in the files: Frequently due to neuroses, often as a sign of apparent "instability", a consequence of negligent (toilet) training, etc.

The fourth most common, with a total of 72 mentions, were "anti-social behaviour, delinquency and neglect". The cases connected to the sexual behaviour of the children and young people were counted separately, in order to show that the cases primarily concerned girls. The fifth place is taken by the so-called psychopathic attributions, which, besides the neurotic attributions, are the most nebulous, but looked back to a long "tradition" in the care and psychiatry of children and young people.[34]

The term "deprivation" in this table was chosen for those cases which are listed in the files as "care damage", but also as (early) neglect or loveless parenting. "Deprivation" does not occur in the files of the examined sample until 1987.

Irrespective of the gender difference, there is the question of why "educational problems" were a reason for psychiatric observation to this extent, as educational problems are not unusual or unexpected. Clearly, the possible consequences of these education problems were considered as being so great that medical clarification was seen as being necessary.

Immediately after the question of "why" comes the question of "who", i.e. who was the driving force between referrals to the unit.

Initiator of referrals

Here, the referring doctors or clinics were not of interest, but rather the actors behind the referrals, who had the greatest interest in the admission of the children to the unit or who were greatly in favour of it. The following groups can be seen in the patient files as the initiators of the referrals:

Tab. 2: Initiators of referrals to the unit between 1949 and 1989

Initiator	Absolute number	Percentage
Parents	196	54.1
Of whom doctors / nerve specialists	34	
Of whom school	14	
Of whom hospital	20	
Of whom other[35]	7	
Youth welfare office/court	97	26.8
Homes	39	10.8
Foster parents	28	7.7
Adoptive parents	2	0.6
Total	362	100

Source: Own calculations

34 In particular, Petra Fuchs has worked on this for period of the Weimar Republic. A new work by her, Wolfgang Rose and Thomas Beddies has just been published, see Rose/ Fuchs/Beddies (2016). Chap. 4. Kinderbeobachtungsstation.

35 These include: Psychological services, education advisory offices, teaching and Kolping homes, child day care facilities.

At 54.1 percent, the parents were in the absolute majority. They have been differentiated between according to the institution giving the parents the advice to send the children to the unit. These also included hospitals, as the parents also had to be in agreement with the referral.

The second most common were offices and authorities at 26.8 percent. Here, the various home facilities (educational homes, orphanages, schools for backward children) and the foster parents were not included, although normally the formal request came from the youth welfare office. This is because the actual initiative came from the appropriate home or foster parents.

Acceptances of the stay costs

The answer to the question of sponsors primarily shows how the stays in the unit were financed, but also offers information on the social care of the natural, adoptive and foster parents of the children and young people.

As the following table shows, of the 362 patients of the child observation unit, it was primarily various health insurers (local health insurance companies, agricultural insurers, railway insurers and company insurers as well state insurance companies for railway and postal workers) who bore the costs of the stay, even in the case of most of the children from Germany and Italy.

Tab. 3: Sponsor of the stay in the child observation station 1949 to 1989

Sponsor	Absolute number	Percentage
Health insurance companies	292	80.6
Private health insurer	22	6.1
No data	22	6.1
Authorities	14	3.9
Did not belong to a health insurer	8	2.2
Direct payer	4	1.1

Source: Own calculations

In the case of at least 14 children and young people (3.9 percent), the costs had to be paid by the authorities (district office, youth welfare office, social security office, social office, district court). It is not known who paid the costs of the 22 children and young people (6.1 percent) for whom there are no details on the sponsor. The same applies to the cases stating that they did not belong to any health insurer. However, overall, it is clear that the group of youngsters for whom the authorities had to act is quite small. In the vast majority of cases, health insurers were obligated to pay. When the authorities had to pay the costs, this often led to very short stays, which was referred to directly in the appropriate cases.

Functions of the unit

In total, it is possible to determine seven functions of the Innsbruck child observation unit.

Its main purpose was to clarify educational, social, "moral", sometimes even legal problems, e.g. theft, with minors and, if possible, to solve them through various therapies.[36] The Innsbruck unit was thus a "hybrid", i.e. did not just observe the children but also gave them therapy, which could also be seen in other units. The very long stays can also be seen in other units and indicate that the appropriate unit made up for the lack of paediatric psychiatric institutions.

If the children no longer seemed to be "sustainable" in their previous location, this usually meant housing in a closed educational home. Many cases dealt with aid in educational issues experienced by parents or foster parents, when they did not know how to handle the child or if a lack of parenting/education in the past had lead to behavioural difficulties.

In addition, the question of cost was important to the authorities. This was the case, for example, if an apparently unfosterable or uneducatable child was in an educational facility. Then, the report of the unit was to determine the inability to be educated, so that the child could be moved to a lower-cost care home.

In the case of girls and boys in family and foster family accommodation, it was for the "protection of society" or the protection of other children and young people that they were moved to an educational home for increased discipline, e.g. if there was a suspicion of "aggressive sexuality".

Easing the workload of the homes was also an important function. It occurred when homes felt overwhelmed with the special circumstances or educational difficulties of certain children and young people and no longer wanted to have to put up with them. In such cases, the unit would look for another accommodation option.

In particular, in the case of children who had already been housed in various homes and with multiple foster families, this had to do with their future place of residence, should the most recent home no longer be regarded as appropriate if the home management or the foster parents no longer wanted the child or if Maria Nowak-Vogl came to the conclusion that the child would be better off elsewhere.

And finally, the unit also offered the option of research and thus an increase in the scientific reputation of the director of qualification of younger operatives. For example, in 1978, a dissertation was written on the recording and treatment of bed-wetting by patients of the Innsbruck unit.[37]

---

36 That simple removal from the previous environment as a so-called "change of scene", i.e. the admission to an observation unit, was said to have a therapeutic benefit should not be forgotten.

37 Cf. Pöhl (1978).

Factors influencing these functions

Here too, multiple aspects are important which cannot always be separated.

The gender and social class of the children and their families of origin were included in no small measure in the examination and could be of significance in the housing of the children after their stay in the unit. A special case were the Yeniche, i. e. the children of the so-called travelling people, to whom a particular character was assigned and who were thus evaluated as limited in their development.

In some cases, the anamnesis was extracted from the behavioural reports of homes or reports of the youth welfare office due to a lack of family members and the prevailing point of view applied to the child, because it was not common practice to question the children and young people themselves when they entered the unit. This means that an unconsidered, written "prejudication" could be the starting point for subsequent observations and would also flow into the final evaluation.

The expectations of the sponsors (youth welfare office, family, foster family) or the parents were certainly taken into account. For example, family members demanded a rapid cure or clarification of the "problems" to aid a speedy discharge. The latter could also be formulated by the authorities, as described above.

"Public opinion" also had an effect. This can be seen in the fact that "preventive" considerations sometimes also flowed into the final evaluation, for example in the case of young people who were to be held back from further thefts, something viewed particularly critically. Here, the educational home was the preferred choice or recommendation.

It is also possible to determine that there were also exceptions, resulting from sympathy and antipathy towards individual children / young people by the head of the unit, irrespective of their class or gender.

Discharge locations of the children

We now turn to the consequential question of where the children went after their stay in the unit. Firstly, we will look at the locations from which the children came to the unit.

Tab. 4: Location of the children before referral to the unit between 1949 and 1989

Location	Absolute number	Percentage
Parents or mother	241	66.6
Grandparents	8	2.2
Aunt/Uncle	4	1.1
Foster parents	43	11.9
Home	49	13.5
Adoptive parents	3	0.8
Other[38]	14	3.9
Total	362	100

Source: Own calculations

As can clearly be seen, at two-thirds of the sample, the group of those coming to the unit from their home is the largest. If other relatives are also included, they make up almost 70 percent. Far behind this, at 13.5 percent, are homes and then foster parents at 11.9 percent. This clearly shows that a stay in the unit was very frequently initiated by the parents/guardians.

The location to which the children were discharged had by far the greatest effect on their lives, both immediately and far beyond. This is shown in the following table:

Tab. 5: Location of the children after discharge from the unit between 1949 and 1989

Locations after discharge fromt the unit	Absolute numbers	Percentage
Parents	208	57.4
Grandparents	9	2.5
Uncle/aunt	4	1.1
Foster parents	33	9.1
Home	73	20.2
Adoptive parents	2	0.6
Escapes	7	1.9
Other	24	6.6
Unknown	2	0.6
Total	362	100

Source: Own calculations

38 These included the children's village, boarding school, trainee/internship with housing, Kolping home, care home.

An absolute majority of the children and young people (57.4 percent) were sent home, followed by to homes (20.2 percent) with foster parents (9.1 percent) in third place. In comparison to Table 4, the location before admission to the unit, it can be seen that homes are more common, whilst the proportion of parents fell back dramatically. This means that almost ten percent of the children did not return to their original family. In the investigated cases, this was frequently due in the interest of the parents or single parents, who felt overburdened with bringing up the child or were no longer interested in the further development of their child. An "override" by the station into an educational home against the will of the parents or guardian occurred only in a very small number of cases. More common in the files is information on resistance by the parents against the official decision for care even before arrival in the unit. The further time progressed, the more statements by youth welfare office representatives increased, showing that there was no desire to be against the wishes of the parents at all costs. The increase in discharges to homes should not detract from the fact that there were also individual cases in which children did not not go back to homes, as Maria Nowak-Vogl was of the opinion that joint education was not good for the appropriate children, or because she found family members willing to take the child.

By the way, the escapes by patients are a phenomenon only found in the last third of the examination sample.

Meaning and consequences of the stay for the children

Firstly, it must be stated that the children and young people were not asked if they wished to go to the unit. Indeed, many of them were not prepared for admission. Under some circumstances, the "transition" to the unit was just as unexpected as the later "transition" to the home, for example. That this had traumatising effects on some children can be seen from interviews with former residents of homes. Some of the former child patients speak today of their traumas, as part of the scandalisation of the unit.

In the best case, the stay in the unit led to help in the form of comprehension, development, explanation, protection or care for the child (and the parents). This did not necessarily mean that children who had been subjected to physical punishment by the parents were housed elsewhere. However, usually, final discussions were held with the parents or guardians, containing information on better education or child development.

The negative consequences of stationary housing could be stigmatisation through the stay, which could possibly be increased by a subsequent stay in a home. Despite the physical separation from the psychiatric clinic, the children of the unit were noticeably psychologically stigmatised. This "label" could make the stigma of being a child in a home even more serious.

Under certain circumstances, the recommendation or specification of the future housing location could have serious consequences on the further development opportunities of the children and young people. Some were taken out of the family without being asked, others were moved to a foster home they had never seen before, yet more had to return to the extremely poor conditions they had come from. The worst cases were referrals to closed educational homes and those to sanatoria and mental hospitals, as, until well into the 1970s, both could mean the end of any development, whilst a stay in a home meant a restriction in individual development.

In general, it is possible to say that character idiosyncrasies or educational errors could create a pathologisation of the child or young person, which could well mark the rest of their lives.

Research outlook

The patient files of the Innsbruck child observation unit, which were handed down in full and are appropriately comprehensive, offer the option of investigating further issues, which have not been tackled so far for reasons of time. Thus, it is possible to present the interdisciplinary work in this unit and the functions of the individual professions in the interplay. Nowak-Vogl said the following of the cooperation between the employees in the Innsbruck unit: "At a weekly four-hour meeting, in which all the employees, i.e. also the teachers, participate, there is a summary report on a child, the result interpreted and the therapy plan for the coming days agreed."[39] Comments on such meetings can be detected regularly in the "course" of the files.

Overall, some basic research must still be carried out, as research into the staff of the paediatric psychiatric profession, with the exception of the psychiatrists, is thin on the ground. The contribution by Maike Rotzoll in this volume shows that paediatric psychiatry was tackled in the theoretical part of the further training of psychiatric nurses. However, its scope and content is as yet unknown.

The correspondence with various institutions (family members, school, youth welfare office, doctor, specialist doctor, court, home, sanatoria and mental hospitals, hospitals), which is handed down in the patient files and some of which is very comprehensive, also allows research to be carried out on the "network", in which the children and young people found themselves.

With regard to nursing history, it can be stated that the field of paediatric psychiatry is an example of the incursion of other professions into an area originally assigned to nursing. For example, care workers also performed nursing tasks during the day, as nurses only worked in the evening. At the beginning, these "care workers" were so-called auxiliary nurses. Some child observation units also talk of kindergarten teachers. Later, graduates and trainees of the Soziale Frauenschule Innsbruck were added[40], who were addressed with "Sister" and their forename and now worked in a psychiatric/remedial

---

39 Vogl (1961), p. 40.
40 The Soziale Frauenschule of the Innsbruck Diocese was founded in 1946.

environment. Some of them also performed psychological tests to ease the work of the psychologists. They had a much closer relationship to the children than the medical and psychological staff. An investigation of this relationship, which can be placed alongside that between the doctor and the patient, has yet to be performed. In addition, their level of involvement in the final diagnosis and prognosis should be determined. Their weekly observation reports could be used for this. It was thus not just the medical staff whose opinion fed into the social construction of a paediatric psychiatric illness, and their influence needs to be researched.

Bibliography

Archival sources

Innsbruck University Archives

Vogl: Denkschrift. Entwicklung der kinderpsychiatrischen Station an der Nervenklinik. 2nd Dec. 1954. Bestand Med. Fakultät, Psychiatrische Kinderstation Sonnenstrasse 44

Tyrolean State Archives, Innsbruck

Patient files of the Innsbruck Paediatric Observation Station

Printed sources

Bleckmann, K.H.: Über die Arbeit einer klinischen Beobachtungsabteilung für erziehungsschwierigen Kinder. In: Praxis der Kinderpsychologie und Kinderpsychiatrie 5 (1956), pp. 8–11.
Emminghaus, H[ermann]: Die psychischen Störungen des Kindesalters. In: Handbuch der Kinderkrankheiten. Edited by Gerhardt, C[arl Adolph Christian Jacob]. Nachtrag II. Tübingen 1887.
Kirmsse, M.: Drei Vorkämpfer der Kinderforschung vor fünfzig Jahren. In: Zeitschrift für Kinderforschung 13 (1908), pp. 307–315.
Müller-Küppers, M.: Aufbau, Funktion und Arbeitsergebnisse (für das Jahr 1961) einer kinderpsychiatrischen Abteilung. In: Praxis der Kinderpsychologie und Kinderpsychiatrie 11 (1962), pp. 167–171.
Pöhl, Ulrich: Ein Beitrag zur Erfassung und Behandlung des Bettnässens. Doctorate, Univ. Innsbruck 1978.
Spiel, W.: 25 Jahre Neuropsychiatrie des Kindes- und Jugendalters in Wien (1951–1976). Supplement to: Zeitschrift für Kinder- und Jugendpsychiatrie 5 (1977) Volume 1.
Stutte, H.: Die Kinder- und Jugendpsychiatrische Station an der Philipps-Universität zu Marburg a.d.L. In: Jahrbuch für Jugendpsychiatrie und ihre Grenzgebiete 2 (1960), pp. 194–202.
Vogl, Maria: Die Kinderpsychiatrische Station des Innsbrucker Krankenhauses. In: Heilpädagogik (1961), p. 38.

Secondary research literature

Beddies, Thomas; Dörries, Andrea (ed.): Die Patienten der Wittenauer Heilstätten in Berlin 1919–1960. Husum 1999.

Buchholz, Matthias: Archivische Überlieferungsbildung im Spiegel von Bewertungsdiskussion und Repräsentativität. 2nd rev. edition, Cologne 2011.

Castell, Rolf et al. (ed.): Geschichte der Kinder- und Jugendpsychiatrie in Deutschland in den Jahren 1937 bis 1961. Göttingen 2003.

Engelbracht, Gerda: Von der Nervenklinik zum Zentralkrankenhaus Bremen-Ost. Bremer Psychiatriegeschichte 1945–1977. Bremen 2004.

Hähner-Rombach, Sylvelyn: "Es ist jetzt das erste Mal, dass ich darüber rede …" Zur Heimgeschichte der Gustav Werner Stiftung zum Bruderhaus und der Haus am Berg gGmbH 1945–1970. Frankfurt/Main 2013.

Hähner-Rombach, Sylvelyn: Routinen psychiatrischer Begutachtung von Kindern und Jugendlichen in einer Beobachtungsstation zwischen 1949 und 1989. In: Taktungen und Rhythmen. Raumzeitliche Perspektiven interdisziplinär (=SpatioTemporality/RaumZeitlichkeit 2). Edited by Schmolinsky, Sabine; Hitzke, Diane; Stahl Heiner. Berlin, Munich [to be published 2017].

Köhnlein, Frank: Zwischen therapeutischer Innovation und sozialer Selektion. Die Entstehung der "Kinderabteilung der Nervenklinik" in Tübingen unter Robert Gaupp und ihre Entwicklung bis 1930 als Beitrag zur Frühgeschichte universitärer Kinder- und Jugendpsychiatrie in Deutschland. Neuried 2001.

Kölch, Michael Gregor: Theorie und Praxis der Kinder- und Jugendpsychiatrie in Berlin 1920–1935. Die Diagnose "Psychopathie" im Spannungsfeld von Psychiatrie, Individualpsychologie und Politik. Med. doct. FU Berlin 2002.

Keim, Ingeborg M.: Die institutionelle Entwicklung der Kinder- und Jugendpsychiatrie in Hessen ab 1900. Frankfurt/Main 1999.

Matron, Kristina: Kommunale Jugendfürsorge in Frankfurt am Main in der Weimarer Republik. Frankfurt/Main 2012.

Orth, Linda: Die Transportkinder aus Bonn: "Kindereuthanasie". Cologne 1989.

Ralser, Michaela: Die Kinderbeobachtungsstation (1954–1987) der Maria Nowak-Vogl und deren Stellung im Fürsorgeerziehungssystem des Landes Tirol. In: Bericht der Medizin-Historischen ExpertInnenkommission: Die Innsbrucker Kinderbeobachtungsstation von Maria Nowak-Vogl. 11th November 2013. (https://www.i-med.ac.at/pr/presse/2013/Bericht-Medizin-Historische-ExpertInnenkommission_2013.pdf, most recently opened on 3.9.2015), p. 28 f.

Rexroth, Christian A. (ed.): Die klinische Kinder- und Jugendpsychiatrie in Bayern. Entwicklungen, Gegenwart, Perspektiven. Commemorative publication on 65th birthday of Dr Martin Linder. Göttingen 2011.

Rose, Wolfgang; Fuchs, Petra; Beddies, Thomas: Diagnose "Psychopathie". Die urbane Moderne und das schwierige Kind. Berlin 1918–1933. Vienna; Cologne; Weimar 2016.

Schaffner-Hänny, Elisabeth: Wo Europas Kinderpsychiatrie zur Welt kam. Anfänge und Entwicklungen in der Region Jurasüdfuss (Aargau, Solothurn, Freiburg, Neuenburg). Dietikon 1997.

Zürrer-Simmen, Susanna: Wege zu einer Kinderpsychiatrie in Zürich. Dietikon 1994.

Deviancy

Theft, Homosexuality, Addiction to Morphium: Cancellation of Diplomas between 1934 and 1965 in Switzerland

Sabine Braunschweig

Summary

The Swiss Central Office for Practical Psychology was responsible for training in psychiatric nursing between 1934 and 1965. The investigation centres on the 27 named diploma cancellations. The Diploma Commission of the Central Office discussed cases of theft, performed abortions, illnesses such as morphine dependency as well as unaccepted behaviour such as homosexuality to determine whether the diploma should be temporary or indefinitely cancelled as a further sanction. Diploma cancellations were part of a range of measures including non-accreditation for training or the final examination, refusal of permanent employment, which were used to keep unsuitable and/or unqualified nurses from plying their trade. This was intended to promote the psychiatric nursing profession and increase the reputation of the psychiatric clinics. Under certain circumstances, it was possible to be given back the diploma after a specified period of time, for example after one year.

Introduction

At the beginning of the 20th century, psychiatric nursing was considered as a menial job without any prestige or competence.[1] It was only when an in-depth course of training was established, in parallel with the professionalisation of psychiatry, that it became a qualified profession. At the end of the 1920s, the Swiss Psychiatric Association (Schweizerische Gesellschaft für Psychiatrie), the professional association of psychiatrists, awarded the first diplomas to psychiatric carers. This meant that, for the first time in Swiss history, at the end of their studies, they were given a certificate confirming their theoretical and practical knowledge of their career field.

This essay concentrates on those psychiatric nurses whose diploma was cancelled. Using various practical case examples, I will indicate the circumstances and areas of conflict which led to the diploma cancellation. It becomes clear ex negativo which standards held sway and what demands were placed on qualified psychiatric personnel.

The topic of diploma cancellations, which belongs to the higher-level question regarding the quality of care and the suitable care personnel, has not previously been investigated in the history of the care-giving professions. There is no suitable research literature.

This work is based on sources which have not yet been evaluated. They are the dossiers of the diploma commission of the Swiss Psychiatric Associa-

---

1 For more information on the professionalisation of psychiatric nursing, cf. Braunschweig (2013), pp. 91–132.

tion. They are in the files of the Swiss Central Office for Practical Psychiatry (Schweizerische Zentralstelle für praktische Psychiatrie), which are stored in the Swiss Social Archives in Zürich. Besides the minutes of the Commission, correspondence on diploma cancellations formed a main source. This runs from 1934, when the Central Office was founded, through to 1965 when it slowly lost its function as a testing and diploma-awarding institution. The files are not complete, meaning that it is not possible to make precise statistical statements. There are 27 names of psychiatric nurses from all over Switzerland who were subject to proceedings.

The development of psychiatric nursing in Switzerland

Until the 1990s, medical care, psychiatric nursing and paediatric nursing care were three distinct professions with their own training, professional associations, periodicals and diplomas. In particular, the following parties were leading lights in the professional development of psychiatric care: The union of psychiatric carers VPOD (Verband des Personals Öffentlicher Dienste), the small professional association for psychiatric nurses and the professional association of psychiatrists.

The sanatoria and mental hospitals showed great deficiencies around 1900: Psychiatric care was poor, the personnel fluctuation high and the reputation of psychiatry in general was low. Reforms were essential. Thus, at the beginning of the 20th century, the VPOD began, on the one hand, to organise the minders in the cantonal sanatoria and mental hospitals and campaigned for better working conditions. On the other hand, individual hospital directors began teaching the minders. Up to that point, they had solely learned from experience. Now, psychiatrists recognised that essential hospital reforms could only be achieved with trained minder personnel. The most prominent figure in the contentual and structural design of the psychiatric care training was the psychiatrist Walter Morgenthaler, who, on the one hand, convinced his psychiatric colleagues of the value of care training and, on the other, was prepared to work together with the union. This resulted in a cooperation, which, though not always harmonious, was successful in the long run, between the Schweizerische Gesellschaft für Psychiatrie and the VPOD as well as smaller staff associations. In 1934, this cooperation resulted in the formation of the Swiss Central Office for Practical Psychiatry, which organised all the issues connected with (further) training as well as job offers and the administrative work of the joint professional periodical.

Morgenthaler made his mark on the training course. In 1922, he created the training programme for the courses, orientated to nursing training courses, formulated the regulations for the examinations, which were held for the first time in 1927, signed the diploma and compiled the instruction manual *Die Pflege der Gemüts- und Geisteskranken*, which was published for the first time in 1930 and was then reissued in seven revised and expanded editions up to

1962. Several editions also appeared in French and Italian and one even in Spanish.

The SGP was thus responsible for the recognition of psychiatric care. In nursing, this was a different matter. With the "Bundesbeschluss vom 25. Juni 1903 betreffend die freiwillige Sanitätshilfe zu Kriegszwecken", the Swiss Red Cross (SRK) had, through successful lobbying in the Swiss federal parliament, been given the competence to manage nursing and monitor training.[2] After the Second World War, the SRK had solidified its role as the leading association for voluntary medical care and nursing to such an extent that it was able to expand this role to paediatric and psychiatric nursing, as well as to all the new non-medical health professions. As many 20th century attempts to integrate the nursing profession into the Swiss Vocational Training Act failed, the SRK was able to adopt this dominant position. Not everyone was happy about this. It took many years of negotiations to reach an agreement between the SRK and the Central Office for Practical Psychiatry, which came into effect on 1st July 1968. From that point on, the SRK was responsible for the recognition of the psychiatric nursing training. Until it was dissolved in 1982, the Central Office continued to deal with questions relating to further training.

As Switzerland has a federal structure and education and health are the responsibility of the cantons, it was therefore not the state that recognised the healthcare professions, but the SRK. However, it was only the agreement of 20th May 1976 between the cantons and the SRK that also regulated this legally and legitimised the function of the SRK as a monitoring body for the healthcare professions.[3]

In 1992, the SRK published the "New training regulations". Now the three specialist training courses in nursing, psychiatric nursing and paediatric and baby nursing were combined into a new general training course in healthcare and nursing, which could be completed at two diploma levels. However, barely 10 years later, the revised federal law of 2002 on professional training and the European "Bologna" educational reform instigated a further training reform. Today, there is a new vocational training course "FAGE" (Fachangestellte Gesundheit – healthcare medical assistant), which can be taken by people over 16. Then, they can study the nursing profession at various levels either at a higher technical college (HF) or at a university of applied sciences (FH). With university entrance examinations from schools, they can then study nursing science at university. This meant that the nursing professions were integrated into the Swiss educational system and are thus controlled by the state. The SRK lost its function.

---

2   For more on the history of nursing, cf. Fritschi (2006). For more on the role of the SRK, cf. Valsangiacomo (1991); Schweikardt (2008), pp. 147–150.
3   Bender (1991), pp. 377–396.

Procedure for diploma cancellation

Until 1940, the hospital commission of the SGP dealt with all issue affecting the training of psychiatric nurses. As the tasks increased, it formed subcommissions, which dealt with issues pertaining to training accreditation, examinations and the textbook.

The Diploma Commission, which, up to that point, had worked independently, was made an independent commission in the revised statutes of the SGP of 1952. "It shall decide on the issue or withdrawal of the nursing diplomas. The chairman and two members are members of the SG. Two further members belong to the staff associations. Election takes place through an open show of hands. The personnel department acts as the secretary and executive organ."[4] Due to this legal formalisation, the commission created a regulation in 1954 as a basis for its work. In the commission meeting, the chairman asked the question of according to which directives decisions were taken when a diploma cancellation was "possible in cases of sickness (e. g. development of mental illness, sexual anomalies, toxicomania) or due to insufficiencies outside work (e. g. immoral behaviour, failed marriage, etc.)".[5] Should the commission try for "schematic regulation" or "give priority to an elastic decision with individual testing of each case"? In the created regulation, Article 5 named the following reasons for diploma cancellation:

  a. In the case of a wanton lifestyle,
  b. In the case of abnormalities of character, leading to a failure in the exercise of their profession or which damage the reputation of the profession,
  c. In the case of a criminal act, even those for which there is no punishment in court,
  d. In the case of serious mental illness.[6]

The procedure for diploma cancellation took place in the following manner: The hospital director or the Central Office itself, if it became aware of a case, could apply to the Diploma Commission to withdraw the diploma of a psychiatric nurse. However, they were obliged first to check the case in detail and clarify it carefully and also to give the appropriate person the opportunity to speak with a member of the Commission.

The five Commission members generally only met once a year for the discussion of basic questions on accreditation for training, the awarding and cancellation of diplomas as well as the resolution of cases, for which no written agreement could be reached. In most cases in the dossier, the members of the Commission agreed unanimously. In some cases, the staff representatives deviated from the majority opinion and asked themselves if there was not

4   Swiss Social Archive (SSA): Ar 31.20.10: Central Office for Practical Psychiatry (Central Office), diploma cancellations, minutes of the Diploma Commission, 20.12.1952.
5   Swiss Social Archive (SSA): Ar 31.20.10: Central Office, diploma cancellations, minutes of the Diploma Commission, 20.12.1952.
6   SSA: Ar 31.20.10: Central Office, diploma cancellations, Regulation of the Diploma Commission of the SGP, Art. 5 (not dated, approx. 1954).

possibly another solution. The diploma could be cancelled for a fixed period of time, for example one year, or indefinitely.

After the decision was taken, the psychiatric nurses were requested to return all the documents to the Central Office. These included the diploma certificate, the brooch and the service book. If the Commission agreed on a temporary diploma cancellation, it also pronounced conditions to be fulfilled to receive the diploma again.

Case studies

The following case studies offer an insight into everyday care work and the working conditions of psychiatric nurses, and show the requirements they had to fulfil in Switzerland in the second third of the 20th century.

Theft

Markus A., born in 1905, had been working as a psychiatric nurse and medical nurse since 1929. By the time he enrolled for the examination in 1938, he had worked in five sanatoriums and asylums. He was recommended by the director of the psychiatric hospital in Basel, who wrote that Markus A. had been working as a private nurse for several weeks for one patient only and had left the hospital with the patient.

> In Mr A., we found an able, attentive, apt and psychologically skilled nurse, to whom we could entrust this very difficult and dangerous patient with a clear conscience. [...] I would give him a "good" grade in practical nursing.[7]

But the director in Basel added that he did not know whether the theoretical and practical knowledge was sufficient for the exam, as Markus A. could not attend the courses regularly. Yet Markus A. passed the exam. When he applied for the diploma one year later, it was refused. It was argued, that he, as an autodidact, did not pass the exam to their satisfaction and the director of the Nervensanatorium Friedheim in Zihlschlacht had not given him a very good reference, and thus he did not receive the diploma.[8] He applied again one year later – this time with a good reference. In the mean time, he worked at the Nervenheilanstalt Schlössli in Oetwil am See. The doctor in charge wrote that A. had behaved well up to that time and had not given any reason for complaint: "He is calm, friendly and skilled in handling patients and very

---

7   SSA: Ar 31.20.10: Central Office, diploma cancellations, case of Markus A.: Letter from Mr Staehelin, director of the Heil- und Pflegeanstalt Friedmatt, Basel, to the Central Office dated 17.2.1938. The forename was changed to make the case anonymous, but the initials were retained.

8   SSA: Ar 31.20.10: Central Office, diploma cancellations, case of Markus A.: Letter from Dr P. Krayenbühl of the Nervensanatorium Friedheim in Zihlschlacht to the Central Office, dated 26.4.1940.

diligent in carrying out his duties. It is fair to say that he is only of middling intelligence, but that is sufficient for his work."[9] Now, Markus A. was awarded the diploma.

After almost two years, the police searched his living accommodation and found clothes, sheets, even a mattress – which, together, was worth 800 Francs, equalling a wage of about 2 months. He had been responsible for the personal belongings of the patients. His former fiancée had denounced him.

The two clinics in which he had most recently worked acted as the plaintiffs. He was "sentenced to 6 months' prison for <u>theft</u> with a conditional deferral of sentence".[10] When the Central Office heard of this, they contacted the director of the Bellevue Clinic in Yverdon in French-speaking Switzerland. He responded that the stolen items had gone unnoticed. When, at the outbreak of the Second World War, Markus A. was drafted into the Swiss Army, the directory gave him a reference which would not negatively affect his future. Markus A. thus received a better reference than he deserved. The director wrote that Markus A. was not integrated into the team of nurses and had the unpleasant habit of continually complaining to the directors. "Whatever is the case, he is culpable for mistakes which should not have happened to a trained nurse, […] which he consistently denied."[11] At the end, everyone was pleased when he left his position early due to mobilisation.

Due to this response and further explanations, the secretary of the Central Office compiled a dossier, which she sent to the chairman of the Diploma Commission with the application for diploma cancellation. In the accompanying letter, she wrote: "After what has happened, M. A. does not seem to us to be suitable for a career in psychiatric nursing and should not be permitted to hold the title of a trained psychiatric nurse."[12] To reinforce this, she stated that he, as an autodidact, only passed the examination with the grade 4.7 [not particularly good] and that the hospital commission had, at first, refused his attempt to obtain a diploma with the requirement that he should complete a further practical year in a recognised hospital. The director of the hospital, from which Markus A. had previously stolen, admitted that he had not signalled the loss to the Central Office out of sympathy, as A. had told him that he had never previously committed theft.[13] The director had thus protected

9   SSA: Ar 31.20.10: Central Office, diploma cancellations, case of Markus A.: Letter from Dr Künzler, Nervenheilanstalt Schlössli, Oetwil am See to Ms Dübi, Central Office, dated 10.9.1941.
10   SSA: Ar 31.20.10: Central Office, diploma cancellations, case of Markus A.: Letter from the Central Office to the medical management of the Nervenheilanstalt Schlössli, Oetwil am See, dated 4.6.1943 (highlighting in original).
11   SSA: Ar 31.20.10: Central Office, diploma cancellations, case of Markus A.: Letter from the Etablissement Bellevue in Yverdon to Ms Dübi, Central Office, dated 21.6.1943.
12   SSA: Ar 31.20.10: Central Office, diploma cancellations, case of Markus A.: Letter from Martha Dübi, Central Office, to Dr Max Müller, Diploma Commission, dated 16.6.1943.
13   SSA: Ar 31.20.10: Central Office, diploma cancellations, case of Markus A.: Letter from Dr H. Künzler, Nervenheilanstalt Schlössli, Oetwil am See to the Central Office, dated 8.6.1943.

him. However, when this director learned of further thefts, he no longer objected to the diploma cancellation measure. At the application of the chairman, the members of the Diploma Commission voted in favour of the sanction.[14]

Theft was not a rare occurrence. A female nurse was dismissed in 1957 because she had stolen large amounts of money out of a colleague's room. When the police and the head nurse searched her room, they found it to be "in total disarray, with a mass of dirty clothes, etc."[15]. It is amazing that the nurse did not fail in her duties, even though her private life was such a catastrophe. The director applied for diploma cancellation. The nurse wished to get married, which, in the 1950s, meant leaving her job, but he was of the opinion that the measure was still adequate, as she had not seemed particularly affected or understanding during the meeting.[16] The diploma cancellation would prevent re-entry into the profession at a later time.

In three further cases of theft, it was not solely the thefts which, besides the dismissal, led to the additional measure of diploma cancellation, but further failings or improper behaviour on the part of the appropriate nurses. One nurse was accused of lying, in addition to being a thief.[17] In 1947, another nurse was "treated in an extremely benevolent manner [...] during her extra-marital pregnancy" and provided with support but was determined to have changed "to her detriment".[18] Rumours were propagated that she "led an immoral lifestyle". When the theft of aprons belonging to a room mate and linen cloths, pillowcases and bathing shirts belonging to the hospital was made known, "this serious crime" and the "character" depravity were no longer compatible "with the ethical code required of a trained nurse". Thus the chairman of the Diploma Commission made the application for diploma cancellation, subject to the condition that she could be given it back if, during a year in a state hospital, she "behaved satisfactorily and the management of this hospital made the application to have the diploma awarded again". The documents do not show if she ever got her diploma back.

14 SSA: Ar 31.20.10: Central Office, diploma cancellations, case of Markus A.: Letter from M. Dübi, Central Office, to Dr Max Müller, Diploma Commission, dated 16.6.1943, with the agreements on the reverse.

15 SSA: Ar 31.20.10: Central Office, diploma cancellations, case of Nina T.: Letter from Prof Dr H. Walther, Kantonale Heil- und Pflegeanstalt Münsingen, to the Central Office, dated 4.5.1957.

16 In the nursing professions, "professional celibacy", i.e. the requirement that they would have to leave the hospital before getting married, existed until the 1950s. The major lack of personnel during the economic boom caused the successive removal of this regulation.

17 SSA: Ar 31.20.10: Central Office, diploma cancellations, case of Danielle M.:

18 SSA: Ar 31.20.10: Central Office, diploma cancellations, case of Esther S., application of the chairman of the Diploma Commission, dated 21.10.1948.

Homosexuality

If the homosexuality of psychiatric nurses was not known or was not visible and caused no problems, then homosexual nurses could work in the profession. Hospital directors had a need for good male nursing personnel and often only intervened when a serious event occurred. Four cases of diploma cancellation were recorded, in which the issue of homosexuality was at the forefront.

Thus, at the end of June 1952, the secretary of the Central Office received a report from the director of the Department of Interior of the Vaud canton (in the French-speaking part of Switzerland) with the request of judgement in the case of Ernest B.[19]

What had happened? Ernest B. was born in 1923 into a peasant family and grew up with four brothers and four sisters. He felt always a little apart and lived quite on his own, as he said later. After he left school, he worked at first on the farm, then he started studies at a school of commerce with the hope of an office job, but the outbreak of World War II prevented him from continuing. So he decided to choose the nursing profession, he learnt psychiatric nursing and was awarded the diploma. Afterwards, he changed to sick-nursing in the state hospital of the canton and went to the nursing school from 1949 to 1951.[20] Shortly before or after his exam in 1951, the following incident occurred. His boyfriend left him, which upset him greatly. After strenuous revision for the sick-nursing exam, he could no longer resist his desires and had an anonymous sexual encounter in a public toilet. The police found him and arrested him. After his release, he hid in his room, did not eat, had suicidal tendencies and was completely devastated.

After a few days absence at his parents' house, he was able to return to the psychiatric clinic in which he had completed his training as a psychiatric nurse and work there.

The director of the Health Office of the Vaud canton asked the Central Office to judge B.'s case. The Health Office would have to check him according to Article 141 of the Cantonal Health Act of 28.9.1928. The question was whether B. should be suspended from his occupation as a nurse or whether this work should be terminated. Article 141 stated:

> If a person in a medical profession, such as a midwife or a nurse, behaves inappropriately, immorally, incapably or negligently in their work, does not fulfil orders or exhibits fraudulent behaviour in public, the government can reprimand him or her, suspend him or her from the profession or even take away the permit to work in the canton.[21]

19   SSA: Ar 31.20.10: Central Office, diploma cancellations, case of Ernest B., letter from the director of Health of the Department of the Interior of the Vaud canton to the Nursing Association and the Central Office, dated 27.6.1952.
20   It was not until the end of the 1940s that male nurses had the opportunity of attending a nursing school recognised by the SRK, cf. Männer in der Krankenpflege Braunschweig (2004).
21   SSA: Ar 31.20.10: Central Office, diploma cancellations, case of Ernest B., copy of Article 141 of the Health Organisation Law of 28.9.1928, the original language being French.

After the Nursing Commission of the Swiss Red Cross had reached a decision not to issue the nursing diploma, in spite of the final examination having been passed successfully, the question arose of what the Central Office for Practical Psychiatry should do.[22] Ernest B. appealed against the refusal of the SRK nursing diploma and wrote that he greatly regretted his transgression.

The chairman of the Diploma Commission, Max Müller, informed the Commission member Georges Schneider, Director of the Cery cantonal psychiatric clinic in Lausanne. Müller wrote

> I think the case needs delicate handling. [...] May I ask you to do something with regard to the case? In accordance with our common practice, we should first give Mr B. the opportunity to speak about his situation and give his opinion on the application for diploma cancellation. As he clearly lives in Lausanne, it would be simplest if you could do this. The minutes of your discussion could then be included in the files for circulation in the Diploma Commission.[23]

The interview took place a few days later, as can be seen in the French-language minutes.[24] The questions that Schneider posed were objective and are testament to a sympathetic attitude. Ernest B.'s answers were accordingly open. When asked how he behaved in the psychiatric clinics and hospitals, he answered that he had always made a strict distinction between a professional relationship and a private relationship. He had never had anything to do with the patients. When informed that his psychiatric nursing diploma might be cancelled, he admitted that he was in a serious situation and that that would not only have moral but also financial consequences.

After that, the psychiatrist wrote in his report that Ernest B. acted like a homosexual, somewhat inhibited with a light stammer, and that he had discovered his homosexuality at 15 or 16. At 22, he had had a "mystic" phase in order to solve his moral problems. It is possible that he left psychiatric nursing in order to avoid delicate situations with patients. After the end of the relationship, he had gone through a depression. He showed no signs of paedophilia. The psychiatrist added that the public prosecutor had led a big campaign against homosexuals. As he could not prosecute all of them, he tried to take administrative sanctions. This was a long process and the culprit was often not kept informed. It was obvious – Schneider wrote – that Ernest B. had damaged the reputation of the nurses by his indecent act, but it was not the expression of a total perversion. Although he was a homosexual, he was proper in his professional work. Schneider advised a temporary diploma cancellation of one year.

---

22   One member of the Commission of the Swiss Red Cross, a psychiatrist, had disclosed that the Red Cross wanted to remove all homosexual nurses from the nursing profession.

23   SSA: Ar 31.20.10: Central Office, diploma cancellations, case of Ernest B.: Letter of the chairman of the Diploma Commission, Prof Dr Max Müller, to Dr G. Schneider, director of the Hôpital de Cery, Lausanne, dated 18.7.1952.

24   SSA: Ar 31.20.10: Central Office, diploma cancellations, case of Ernest B., minutes of the interview between Dr G. Schneider with Ernest B., dated 22.7.1952.

When the members of the Commission discussed the case, they emphasised that they did not want to punish his homosexuality but only the special
incident happening in the public and that they wanted to protect the reputation of the nursing profession.[25] They felt themselves to be in a dilemma and
under pressure because the commission of the Swiss Red Cross had acted so
quickly, drastically and irrevocably. Because, at that time, the Swiss Psychiatric
Association and the Swiss Red Cross had started negotiations about the recip-
rocal recognition of both formations of sick-nursing and psychiatric nursing,
the psychiatrists felt uneasy to take another position to that of the Swiss Red
Cross.

Finally, the members of the Diploma Commission agreed on the cancellation of the diploma for one year and added the warning that Ernest B. would
lose the diploma immediately and indefinitely if he ever behaved improperly
with patients.[26] However, the union representative was not happy with this
decision as B. had never actually been in trouble in the course of his professional work.[27]

The Swiss parliament had dealt with the new Penal Code from 1929 onwards. The question of homosexuality and its culpability was particularly controversial. Criminal lawyers and psychiatrists argued for the exemption from
punishment for homosexual activities, because new studies had produced new
awareness about the nature of homosexuality. The Swiss Penal Code, which
finally took effect in 1942, did instigate the decriminalisation of homosexuality, but now its interpretation as a mental illness increased, along with the
question of whether it could be treated.[28] This was a consequence of the increased influence of the medical and psychiatric viewpoint.[29]

Compared to the old cantonal penal codes and the international situation,
the Swiss Penal Code was quite liberal in this respect. Nevertheless, there were
conservative politicians, doctors and lawyers who followed a hard line against
homosexuals as the majority in the Nursing Commission of the Swiss Red
Cross had shown.

25 SSA: Ar 31.20.10: Central Office, diploma cancellations, case of Ernest B., letter of the
    chairman Max Müller to Payot, director of the Health Office, dated 15.8.1952.
26 SSA: Ar 31.20.10: Central Office, diploma cancellations, case of Ernest B., letter of the
    chairman Max Müller to Ernest B., dated 15.8.1952.
27 SSA: Ar 31.20.10: Central Office, diploma cancellations, case of Ernest B., response of
    Walter Vollenweider, VPOD, 12.8.1952.
28 Only male prostitution and sexual intercourse between men below the age of 20 years
    remained criminal acts. Cf. Walser, Erasmus: Homosexualität, in: Historisches Lexikon
    der Schweiz (HLS), http://www.hls-dhs-dss.ch/textes/d/D16560.php (27.6.2016).
29 It was not until 1991 that homosexuality was removed as a psychiatric diagnosis from the
    international statistical classification of illness and related health problems (ICD-10) pub-
    lished by the WHO.

After the period of a year had elapsed, Ernest B. requested the return of his diploma. As there had been no negative occurrences, he received his diploma, service book and identity card back.[30]

During the same period, the Vaud Department of Health decreed that the nurse Eric R. should have his permission to work rescinded for one year. R. was sentenced to 45 days in prison with a probational period of two years as he had had sexual contact with a young prisoner who had been in the psychiatric clinic for observation.[31]

However, the Diploma Commission had already cancelled the diploma for an indefinite period of time and suggested that he take up a post in a geriatric home.[32] The lawyer of the nurse had submitted an appeal against the decision of the Diploma Commission. Nonetheless, the members unanimously stuck to their application for diploma cancellation, but were prepared to review the case after the two-year probational period. R. needed the diploma to perform his work, as the healthcare authorities could only issue the authorisation to work to nursing staff with a diploma. Even if they prevented him from working for one year, they could not permit him to do it again for as long as he had not had his diploma returned.

After the two-year probational period, Eric R. again attempted to obtain the issue of his diploma and also sent an extract of the criminal register. The crime had been deleted from it. He wrote that he had been on night watch for two years with an elderly man and now, for financial reasons, wished to work as a trained carer. He had two children who were treated in Leysin for tuberculosis. As nothing detrimental had come to light about Eric R. over the last two years, the Diploma Commission was in agreement that he should receive his diploma back again.[33]

Addictions

The risk of addiction in the nursing profession was high.[34] The deputy head nurse of a psychiatric hospital, the 30-year-old nurse Lina G., had become addicted to morphine in the 1940s. As nurses had the key to the medicine cupboard, they sometimes helped themselves to solve their own problems. Addiction to painkillers was a known problem among nurses and doctors.

The director of the hospital who found out about her addiction was asked by the Diploma Commission to apply for a cancellation of the diploma. He wrote that Lina G. had worked as deputy head nurse from the autumn of 1939

---

30 SSA: Ar 31.20.10: Central Office, diploma cancellations, case of Ernest B., return of the diploma and other documents to Ernest B., dated 28.8.1954.

31 SSA: Ar 31.20.10: Central Office, diploma cancellations, case of Eric R.

32 SSA: Ar 31.20.10: Central Office, diploma cancellations, case of Eric R., cf. minutes of the Diploma Commission, dated 24.9.1955.

33 SSA: Ar 31.20.10: Central Office, diploma cancellations, case of Eric R., cf. minutes of the Diploma Commission, dated 24.9.1955.

34 Cf. occupation-dependent illnesses in nursing professions Braunschweig (2012).

until the end of 1943.[35] He was not sure if she had already been addicted at her previous place of work. At the end of 1942, she got an abscess on her thigh. When she was infected several times, the surgeon assumed that these abscesses came from an infection of injections. The director had asked her about this a few times, but she denied it. Only in December 1943 could he provide evidence that she had taken morphine and Pantopon pills. When she realised that she had no other alternative, she admitted it all.

The director added that he was able to show the cantonal Department of Health that Lina G. was not involved in a criminal investigation but that she had been regarded "from the start as a certifiable addict". He had arranged for her to be moved to a private clinic in another canton. Both he and the clinic doctors had told her she should give up her work immediately. However, she ignored this advice and left the clinic after two months. The director characterised Lina G. as a very pleasant, healthy woman who was quite talented in handling the patients, thanks to her cheerful and nice way. But, after a while, he noticed that she had become more and more cursory, had less patience in her work and showed ill humour. He did not see any symptoms of schizophrenia but he noticed the common attitude of addicts pretending they could stop at once if they wanted. She had lost the feeling for the egregious way she had abused his confidence and how shamelessly she had been lying. Although he did not have a lot of experience with toxicomanias, he gave a bad prognosis. Therefore, he approved the cancellation of her diploma.

After Lina G. had terminated her detoxification programme and had left the private clinic, she found a job in a sanatorium. However, she relapsed within one month. Her superior found out that she used injections intended for a patient on herself. The cantonal Department of Health was now informed, leading to the process of diploma cancellation. Firstly, the head of the Healthcare Directorate informed the professional association to which Lina G. belonged that he did not yet want "a general suspension of the procurement of anaesthetics by all cantonal governments". He did, though, wish to prevent "this nurse from carrying on this nursing work, which was dangerous to her, and each hospital from having to discover for itself that toxicomania existed".[36]

The professional association contacted Lina G. and submitted a report to the Healthcare Directorate. The chairman wrote: Lina G. had, "after pressure from us", decided to temporarily refrain from practising nursing for a period of at least one year. She would look for work in a household or return to her previous profession as a saleswoman in the textiles industry. Until that time, the professional association would wait with exclusion and diploma cancella-

35 SSA: Ar 31.20.10: Central Office, diploma cancellations, case of Lina G., letter from the director of the Heil- und Pflegeanstalt Münsterlingen, A. Zolliker, to the chairman of the Diploma Commission, Prof Dr Max Müller, 9.10.1944.

36 SSA: Ar 31.20.10: Central Office, diploma cancellations, case of Lina G., letter from the Healthcare Directorate, H. Büchel, to the chairman of the Schweizerischer Verbandes der Pflegerinnen für Nerven- und Gemütskranke, Dr Friedrich Braun, dated 3.8.1944.

tion and, after the probational period, would demand "a further period of observation and quarantine of approx. three to four weeks in a mental hospital". If her addiction resurfaced, then the professional association would not waste any time in taking all the named measures.[37] The professional association informed the Central Office of this.[38] The keen secretary at the Central Office contacted the chairman of the Diploma Commission as to whether it was wise to wait with an application for diploma cancellation and whether further information should not be gained from earlier places of work.[39] The chairman was pessimistic: "I have little hope in this situation that a period of grace of one year will actually achieve anything. I am more of the opinion that the person concerned should leave the nursing profession without delay."[40] However, as an application for diploma cancellation had to be made, he suggested obtaining further information from the director that discovered the situation and to ask him if he would make such an application. As was mentioned at the beginning, the latter stated that he had to bring himself to make this application: "After considerable consideration, I see that, as I view the situation, I have no alternative but to request diploma cancellation."[41] This complex formulation showed that it was not easy for him.

Now the members of the Diploma Commission indicated that they supported the diploma cancellation. Lina G. decided not to appeal and finally returned all the identification documents.[42]

In cases of addiction, psychiatrists were somewhat sceptical of whether a temporary sanction could "wean" psychiatric nurses off their addiction. This was expressed in a letter by the director of the Heil- und Pflegeanstalt Münsingen (Berne canton), who was applying for a diploma cancellation. This was to do with the case of Erna B. who, at the beginning of 1961, was sent to the hospital for clarification "of an opiate addiction with psychopathic development".[43] Erna B. had become addicted to morphine in 1955, left her post in a psychiatric hospital, worked for two years at a dentist's and then in a hospital – lastly on night watch in a surgical ward. Her addiction to medicines such as

37 SSA: Ar 31.20.10: Central Office, diploma cancellations, case of Lina G., letter from Dr F. Braun, Association chairman, to the Health Directorate, dated 28.8.1944.

38 SSA: Ar 31.20.10: Central Office, diploma cancellations, case of Lina G., letter of the Schweizerischer Verband der Pflegerinnen für Nerven- und Gemütskranke to the Central Office, dated 1.9.1944.

39 SSA: Ar 31.20.10: Central Office, diploma cancellations, case of Lina G., letter from the Central Office to the chairman of the Diploma Commission, dated 30.9.1944.

40 SSA: Ar 31.20.10: Central Office, diploma cancellations, case of Lina G., letter of the chairman of the Diploma Commission, dated 2.10.1944.

41 SSA: Ar 31.20.10: Central Office, diploma cancellations, case of Lina G., letter from the director of the Heil- und Pflegeanstalt Münsterlingen, A. Zolliker, to the chairman of the Diploma Commission, Prof Dr Max Müller, 9.10.1944.

42 SSA: Ar 31.20.10: Central Office, diploma cancellations, case of Lina G., return by Lina G. to the Central Office, dated 30.4.1945.

43 SSA: Ar 31.20.10: Central Office, diploma cancellations, case of Erna B., letter from the director of the cantonal Heil- und Pflegeanstalt Münsingen to the Diploma Commission, dated 13.3.1961.

dolantine, pethidiane and Vilan was noticed in the autumn of 1960, which she readily admitted. She wanted to undergo "rehabilitation treatment", but left the hospital after only a brief time. In his letter, the director characterised her as follows: "The personality of the patient is psychopathic. She is intelligent but defiant, closed and impenetrable, shallow, compulsive and opportunistic."[44] He gave her an unpromising prognosis, in spite of the fact that her relatives supported her "in her obstinacy". He applied to the Health Directorate to place Erna B. on a black list "as the addict should not be active in the nursing profession if she cannot be permanently treated for her addiction". In his opinion, the diploma cancellation could be condition, subject to her "further rehabilitating under medical supervision and subsequently submitting to examinations over a long term period". He was sure that she would not accept this condition but that he had at least given her the chance of not losing her diploma permanently.

The Diploma Commission voted four to one in favour of a diploma cancellation.[45] The one vote against was that of the MP Karl Geissbühler, a member of the Social Democratic Party. The representative of the Berne State Personnel Association had spoken to Erna B. She informed him that she had given up her nursing career and had stopped taking all opiates of her own accord. Treatment was not necessary. She was attending a private commercial school and hoped to be awarded her diploma soon.[46]

Abortion

The dossier on diploma cancellations also contains files on two psychiatric nurses who performed abortions. The director of the Hospice de Perreux discovered in May 1956 that, six months after completing his training, the 28 year-old Julien F. had performed an abortion on a young waitress in one of the pavilions within the clinic grounds and had demanded a "fee of CHF 300".[47] The director informed the public prosecutor of the Neuenburg (Neuchâtel) canton, who instigated criminal proceedings. The nurse admitted the charges and also tried to draw a doctor and another nurse into the matter. The director wrote that F. was no longer "worthy" of a diploma and applied for diploma cancellation.

---

44   SSA: Ar 31.20.10: Central Office, diploma cancellations, case of Erna B., letter from the
     director of the cantonal Heil- und Pflegeanstalt Münsingen to the Diploma Commission,
     dated 13.3.1961.
45   SSA: Ar 31.20.10: Central Office, diploma cancellations, case of Erna B., letter from the
     Central Office to the chairman of the Diploma Commission, dated 29.4.1961.
46   SSA: Ar 31.20.10: Central Office, diploma cancellations, case of Erna B., letter from
     Geissbühler to the Diploma Commission, dated 27.3.1961.
47   SSA: Ar 31.20.10: Central Office, diploma cancellations, case of Julien F., letter from the
     director of the Hospice de Perreux, Dr de Montmollin, to the chairman of the Diploma
     Commission, dated 16th May 1956.

The chairman wrote to his colleagues in the Diploma Commission, saying that he agreed to a temporary cancellation and that the definitive decision should be taken after the criminal investigation had been completed.[48] Two of the contacted members took a hard line and approved an immediate diploma cancellation without waiting for the result of the criminal investigation, particularly as the nurse had admitted the crime. The two other employees supported the chairman.

When it was requested, Julien F. returned the diploma, the service book and the identification, but was apparently unable to find the silver badge and the five fabric badges. The documents do not show whether the discussion he requested in his accompanying letter actually took place.[49] However, he had already found a new job in an industrial company, which was not difficult during the economic boom and the lack of workers.[50]

Conclusions

As no statistical figures are available on the diplomas awarded, these 27 named cases cannot be evaluated statistically. It was not until 1956 that the Central Office was given the task of preparing annual statistics on the training courses. Only information on the total number of people examined in 1943 could be found in the sources. According to those statistics, 2,403 candidates had been examined between the start of examinations in 1927 and 1943. How many of them had not received the diploma after a further year in work is not stated.[51] Due to the missing statistical figures, it is not currently possible to make a statement on how many psychiatric nurses received the diploma between 1927, when the first examinations were held, and 1968 when the agreement with the SRK took effect. It can be assumed that the cases of diploma cancellation found made up barely half of one percent of all the diplomas awarded. Thus, the one or two cases per year represent exceptions. They did not pose a central problem in the professional development of psychiatric nursing.

48 SSA: Ar 31.20.10: Central Office, diploma cancellations, case of Julien F., letter from chairman Georg Stutz, director of the Hasenbühl in Liestal, to the Diploma Commission, dated 20.6.1956.

49 SSA: Ar 31.20.10: Central Office, diploma cancellations, case of Julien F., letter from Julien F. to the secretary of the Central Office, dated 28.1.1957.

50 SSA: Ar 31.20.10: Central Office, diploma cancellations, case of Julien F., letter from Câbles Cortaillod to the Central Office, dated 5.2.1957.

51 SSA: Ar 31.20.10: Central Office, annual report 1943.

Tab. 1: Cases of diploma cancellation

Transgression or "incorrect behaviour"	Male psychiatric nurses	Female psychiatric nurses
Theft	2	3
"Morality crime" (homosexual behaviour)	4	0
Addictions	0	4
Abortion performed	2	
Psychiatric diagnosis (e. g. epilepsy)	0	2
Reasons not known	2	8
Total	10	17

Of the 27 cases of diploma cancellation, 10 concerned male psychiatric nurses and 17 concerned female psychiatric nurses. They provide certain indications of which transgressions and behaviours could lead to a temporary or indefinite diploma cancellation. In the case of thefts, which occurred frequently, an additional reason was required before this serious sanction was taken. In the cases found, these included a lack of remorse and lies. Homosexuality was only of significance amongst male nurses and usually accompanied temporary diploma cancellations. Addictions such as "opiate and morphine addiction" and drug abuse were forms of expression specific to women. Five diploma cancellations occurred in German-speaking Switzerland and five in French-speaking Switzerland, whilst one male nurse worked in both sections of the country. In 10 cases, only the names are known but there is no further information on the transgressions and places of work. Only three cases document what the nurse did after diploma cancellation. One psychiatric nurse got married, another went abroad and one male nurse worked in an industrial company. After diploma cancellation, it was possible to work as an assistant in nursing, as is shown in the case of one male nurse, who worked as a night watchman in a private hospital during the period of his temporary diploma cancellation. However, this represented a major financial blow.

Even if these diploma cancellations are not significant in terms of actual numbers, in the context of the professional development of psychiatric care, then they form a piece of the mosaic of the question of the quality of care and nursing in psychiatric hospitals. For the Diploma Commission, the explanations on the accreditation for training and examination, on the issue or withdrawal of the diploma were used "in the interest of the profession [...] to draw in as many qualified carers as possible".[52] The topic of the quality of care had driven the mental doctors and psychiatrists since the psychiatric reforms in the second half of the 19th century. The improvement in working conditions, such as increased wages, approval of living outside the hospital or the permis-

---

52   SSA: Ar 31.20.10: Central Office, Diploma Commission, minutes of 20.9.1952.

sion to get married were no longer sufficient to recruit trained, reliable care personnel. When the new somatic cures appeared in the 1920s and 1930s, qualified assistants were essential.

Whilst some hospital directors feared that "half-trained" minders would challenge their authority when the first courses were introduced, others recognised the necessity of training the psychiatric care staff. Questions of selection were commonplace – along with the dilemma of promoting the profession against supporting those already working in it. The training pioneer Morgenthaler described this dichotomy as follows: "How can two such different masters be served: On the one hand, the strict removal of all those deemed unsuitable, the improvement of the business as a whole, the training of the staff into as perfect a precision instrument as possible and aid for the main task of the hospital and, on the other hand, the human requirement for mutual aid, particularly aid to and support of those with fewer or few skills?"[53]

The "psychotechnical methods", developed in Germany in the early 20th century, which were seen as the method of the future for evaluating the character and ability of workers, were also discussed in Switzerland. Could "psychotechnology" be used to determine the suitability of candidates in nursing? Morgenthaler evaluated the technically complex methods which Fritz Giehse, Head of the Institute for Practical Psychology in Halle an der Saale, had devised as being too lengthy and too complex. He did not exclude a small psychotechnical examination, but he was "against shallow and uncompromising psychotechnical examinations".[54] This opinion was shared by other renowned Swiss psychiatrists, such as Charlot Strasser, who, as a socialist and anti-fascist, expressed critical views on various psychiatric subjects.[55]

When looking through these cases of diploma cancellation, I – in conclusion – cannot rid myself of the impression that it was fairly random whether a nurse was involved in such a process or not. In countless personnel dossiers from the Basel Heil- und Pflegeanstalt Friedmatt which I viewed, similar cases occur which, however, never led the director to apply for diploma cancellation. The supervisory commission at Friedmatt also never suggested a diploma cancellation as a sanction. The psychiatric nurse who had stolen the linen cloths, towels and dresses was dismissed and was forced to return the stolen items. She had to pay damages for those items of clothing she had already cut up and modified. Thefts kept occurring and it was impossible to prevent them from doing so, said the chairman of the Commission pragmatically. This case too had only come to light due to the denunciation.[56] The psychiatric nurse who had abused a patient was dismissed and sentenced to two months in

---

53   Morgenthaler (1933), p. 136. Cf. Braunschweig (1988), p. 92 f.
54   Morgenthaler (1934); Giehse (1924). On psychotechnology: Messerli (1996), Braunschweig (1988), p. 92.
55   Heinrich (1986).
56   Staatsarchiv Basel-Stadt (StABS): Health files T2, 1886–1933: Friedmatt, minutes of the Supervisory Commission, dated 3.4.1929.

prison with a 5-year probational period. Diploma cancellation was not at issue.[57]

Clearly, similar cases of misconduct by nursing staff in various psychiatric hospitals were penalised, although in different manners. And clearly not all hospital doctors wished to make the punishment even stricter through a diploma cancellation, making the opportunities of the person to obtain employment in future even worse.

As most employees in the first decades of the 20th century lived in the hospital complex, the doctors knew the nursing staff better, knew a lot about their private lives, knew their strengths and weaknesses and thus had more understanding for their transgressions.

By contrast, the Swiss Central Office for Practical Psychiatry was obliged to promote the profession and was extremely keen to eliminate nursing staff considered as "unsuitable". Further research in this field would be interesting to look into the question of selection and randomness in sanctions. Case examples could show further which social norms and requirements were required of nursing staff and with which sanctions transgressions were punished.

Bibliography

Archival sources

Swiss Social Archive (SSA):

Ar 31.20.10: Swiss Central Office for Practical Psychiatry (Central Office): Dossiers: Annual
    reports, correspondence on diploma cancellations, minutes of the Diploma Commission.

Staatsarchiv Basel-Stadt (StABS):

Health files T2, 1886–1933: Friedmatt, minutes of the Supervisory Commission.

Printed sources

Giehse, Fritz: Psychotechnische Verfahren für Pflegepersonal in Heilanstalten. In: Zeitschrift
    für die gesamte Neurologie und Psychiatrie 88 (1924), pp. 533–549.
Morgenthaler, Walter: Bildung und Ausbildung beim schweizerischen Pflegepersonal für
    Gemüts- und Geisteskranke, (Personal- und Anstaltsfragen 7) Berne 1934.
Morgenthaler, Walter: Das Problem der Durchgefallenen. In: Kranken- und Irrenpflege 7
    (1933), pp. 134–138.

---

57 Braunschweig (2013), pp. 157–161.

Secondary research literature

Bender, Philippe: Entstehung und Inhalt der Vereinbarung vom 20. Mai 1976. In: Valsangiacomo, Enrico (ed.): Zum Wohle der Kranken. Das Schweizerische Rote Kreuz und die Geschichte der Krankenpflege. Basel 1991, pp. 377–396.

Braunschweig, Sabine: Zwischen Aufsicht und Betreuung. Berufsbildung und Arbeitsalltag der Psychiatriepflege am Beispiel der Basler Heil- und Pflegeanstalt Friedmatt, 1886–1960. Zürich 2013.

Braunschweig, Sabine: Wenn Psychiatriepflegende selbst erkranken. Pflegekrisen im Alltag einer psychiatrischen Anstalt in den 1930er Jahren. In: Traverse 2 (2012), pp. 57–67.

Braunschweig, Sabine: Auf den Spuren der Männer in einem Frauenberuf – weshalb die Krankenpflege weiblich ist. In: Bosshart-Pfluger, Catherine; Grisard, Dominique; Späti, Christina (ed.): Geschlecht und Wissen? Genre et savoir? Gender and Knowledge? Zürich 2004, pp. 123–130.

Braunschweig, Sabine: hüten – warten – pflegen. Das Pflegepersonal der Heil- und Pflegeanstalt Friedmatt in Basel, Basel 1988 (unpublished Master thesis).

Fritschi, Alfred: Schwesterntum. Zur Sozialgeschichte der weiblichen Berufskrankenpflege in der Schweiz 1850–1930. 2nd ed. Zürich 2006.

Heinrich, Daniel: Dr. med. Charlot Strasser (1884–1950). Ein Psychiater als Schriftsteller, Sozial- und Kulturpolitiker. Zürich 1986.

Messerli, Jakob: Psychotechnische Rationalisierung. Zur Verwissenschaftlichung von Arbeit in der Schweiz im frühen 20. Jahrhundert. In: Pfister, Ulrich; Studer, Brigitte; Tanner, Jakob (ed.): Arbeit im Wandel. Organisation und Herrschaft vom Mittelalter bis zur Gegenwart. Zürich 1996, pp. 233–258.

Schweikardt, Christoph: Zur Berufsgeschichte der Pflege in der Schweiz. In: Hähner-Rombach, Sylvelyn (ed.): Quellen zur Geschichte der Krankenpflege. Frankfurt/Main 2008, pp. 147–150.

Valsangiacomo, Enrico (ed.): Zum Wohle der Kranken. Das Schweizerische Rote Kreuz und die Geschichte der Krankenpflege. Basel 1991.

Walser, Erasmus: Homosexualität. In: Historisches Lexikon der Schweiz: http://www.hls-dhs-dss.ch/textes/d/D16560.php.

"Heroic Theapies" and Nursing

"Shock Therapies" and Nursing in the Psychiatric Clinic of the University of Würzburg in the 1930s and 1940s[1]

Karen Nolte

Summary

In the middle of the 1930s German psychiatrists began to treat patients who had been diagnosed with schizophrenia with the new shock therapies: insulin shock and metrazol shock therapy (in German Cardiazolkrampftherapie). In the 1940s electroconvulsive treatment was initially also used to treat patients with schizophrenia. This article analyses the nursing practice that accompanied these new somatic therapies, drawing on the example of the Psychiatric and Neurological Hospital at the University of Würzburg (Psychiatrische und Nervenklinik der Universität Würzburg).[2] While the everyday nursing routine was not documented in the department of psychiatry and can only be indirectly deduced from the doctors' notes in the patient records, the nurses' notes on insulin shock therapy are available in the files on special charts for this treatment. I will historically contextualise these handwritten notes by the nurses and analyse them together with the patient records in which we can find traces of the nurses' actions in between the lines.

Introduction

In the middle of the 1930s new somatic therapies were introduced in German psychiatry departments. The insulin shock therapy had been developed by the Polish doctor Manfred Sakel (1900–1957) between 1933–1935 at the university hospital in Vienna where he tested it in schizophrenics. Already in 1935 this therapy was used for the first time in the Hospital of Psychiatric and Mental Disorders at the University of Gießen on 15 schizophrenic patients. According to the notes, in "fresh" cases of schizophrenia a "remarkably quick remission" had been achieved and even "prolonged schizophrenic processes" had been positively influenced.[3] Until the end of 1936 this new somatic therapy had been adopted by 34 additional psychiatric institutions.[4] At the beginning of 1936 the Hospital of Psychiatric and Mental Disorders at the University of Würzburg also began some first attempts to treat schizophrenic patients

---

1   A very heartfelt thank you goes to Prof. Dr. Jürgen Deckert who went to great pains to ensure that historians would gain access to the archives of patient records at the University Psychiatric Hospital that is today called "Zentrum für psychische Gesundheit" (Centre for Psychological Health).
2   In 1939 the "Psychiatric and Neurological Hospital at the University of Würzburg" was renamed into "University Psychiatric Hospital Würzburg."
3   Cf. Hamann-Roth (1999), p. 25. The quotes are by Wilhelm Ederle (1901–1966) who conducted these therapy trials on his own in Gießen, cited after Hamann-Roth (1999), p. 25.
4   Cf. Beyer (2013), p. 233.

with the new insulin shock therapy.[5] The prominent German psychiatric-neu-rological journals were full of publications in which German psychiatrists – largely euphorically – reported about their own therapeutic trials, especially in the first years after Sakel's publication.[6] Yet, the scientific interest in Würzburg seems to have been very low. While nearly all German university hospitals published about their experiences with Sakel's therapy, contributions by the psychiatrists in Würzburg cannot be found. The Hospital of Psychiatric and Mental Disorders at the University of Würzburg is only mentioned once in an "Overview over the cases of schizophrenia treated according to the method of the Viennese Psychiatric Hospital (hypoglycaemia shock)" ("Über-sicht über die nach der Methode der Wiener Psychiatrischen Klinik (Hypo-klykämie-Chok) behandelten Schizophreniefälle"), stating that it had treated three cases in 1936.[7] The dissertations in psychiatry submitted in Würzburg after 1936 do not address the insulin shock therapy either so that we can as-sume that there was very little scientific interest in this new form of therapy at the hospital in Würzburg.[8] Nonetheless this therapy was used early – albeit rarely – in schizophrenic patients.[9]

Metrazol shock therapy by contrast, which the Hungarian psychiatrist Ladislaus Meduna (1896–1964)[10] had developed, was used quite often in Würzburg in schizophrenic patients, and at times also in combination with insulin shock therapy. Originating from the idea that there is an antagonism between epilepsy and schizophrenia, the artificially created epileptic convul-sion was thought to have a healing effect in psychotic and catatonic schizo-phrenia. In Würzburg this therapy was already practised in the year when Meduna's scientific results of his therapeutic trials with metrazol shock ther-

---

5   Sakel (1935).
6   I systematically reviewed the following journals for the years 1936–1941: Psychia-trisch-Neurologische Wochenschrift, Der Nervenarzt, Allgemeine Zeitschrift für Psychia-trie and the Deutsche Zeitschrift für Nervenheilkunde.
7   Übersicht über die nach der Methode der Wiener Psychiatrischen Klinik (Hypogly-kämie-Chok) behandelten Schizophreniefälle. In: Psychiatrisch-Neurologische Wochen-schrift 35 (1936), p. 423.
8   Cf. especially Thumm (1938). This literature review on the insulin and metrazol treat-ment does not contain any reference to research in Würzburg. Most articles on the topic were published between 1936 and 1938. Cf. also the research report by Oberholzer (1940). Only in 1942 the Allgemeine Zeitschrift für Psychiatrie und ihre Grenzgebiete published a study by the Würzburg psychiatrist Rudolf Tangermann who used patient records of the sanatorium and nursing home Werneck from the years 1925–1934 to ex-amine spontaneous remissions in schizophrenia and to compare these numbers with figures on remissions in the centres that had used the insulin shock therapy (Cf. Tanger-mann, 1942).
9   At the Institute for the History of Medicine at the University of Würzburg I discovered the estate of Professor Dr. Martin Reichardt who owned a large collection of special re-search publications. These journals and articles reveal more about the focus of research at the University Psychiatric Hospital under Reichardt (1925–1939), which was in par-ticular research on psychiatric and neurological assessment of accidents and brain re-search. There are only very few special editions on shock therapies.
10   Meduna (1937).

apy were published in German.[11] Yet the scientific interest in this therapy was also quite low: there are no publications by Würzburg psychiatrists in the known psychiatric journals nor are there any dissertations on the topic from Würzburg. Electroconvulsive treatment was developed by the Italians Ugo Cerletti (1877–1963) and Lucio Bini (1908–164) and initially tested at the university hospital in Rome. In Germany it was used for the first time in 1939 in Erlangen when the psychiatrist Friedrich Meggendorfer (1880–1953) collaborated with the company Siemens to use it to treat schizophrenics. In Würzburg this new somatic therapy was introduced in 1940 and used to treat schizophrenics but also in patients with depression.

As Sabine Braunschweig established in her research on the history of psychiatric care in Switzerland, the nursing staff was crucial for the introduction and establishment of new somatic therapies as the patients required careful monitoring.[12]

For this article I rely on the patient records from the Psychiatric and Neurological Hospital at the University of Würzburg as the source for my analysis of the nursing practice in this subfield of psychiatric therapy. I show how the shock therapies changed the psychiatric everyday experience and how that change had an impact on the work of the nursing staff. The doctor's notes in the patient records were mainly based on the oral and written reports about the everyday experiences at the ward that the nursing staff provided. The original reports by the nurses about the behaviour of the patients and events on the ward were not added to the patient records because they had become part of the doctors' entries. Hence they might not have been regarded as worth keeping. In the manual on the *Pflege der Gemüts- und Geisteskranken* (Care of Psychological and Mental Patients) from 1930 by the Swiss psychiatrist Walter Morgenthaler (1882–1965) there is only one explicit instruction for nurses on how to monitor patients and in what form and at what time these observations had to be reported to the doctor.[13] Sabine Braunschweig has illustrated how doctors' notes about the patients' behaviour can be read against the grain to reconstruct the original observations of the nurses.[14] The exception were the patient records of those treated with insulin shock therapy as here we find notes that had indeed been written by the nurses themselves. For a successful insulin shock therapy the nurses' thorough documentation of the measurements and physical symptoms on the one hand, and their observations of the behaviour and the patient's psychological well-being on the other hand, was absolutely vital. For that reason these sources will be analysed more closely in this article.

In the following I will extract the carers' observations from the doctors' notes and also analyse the reports available that the nurses had written themselves. Which entries did the doctors copy into the notes and which observa-

---

11 Meduna (1937).
12 Cf. Braunschweig (2013), pp. 197–202.
13 Morgenthaler (1930), pp. 151–162.
14 Cf. Braunschweig (2013), pp. 182–184.

tions did they receive from carers who did not write them themselves into the patient records? Another question is whether the kind of written documentation reveals a hierarchy of tasks among the carers.

Sources

The sources are extraordinarily numerous and rich with regards to the patient history and aspects of everyday history. Since the hospital's foundation in 1893 until today nearly all of the patient records have survived, discounting normal loss due to everyday wear and tear. For the period between 1936–1945 alone, there should be approximately 10,000 files – a figure I estimate from the number of available admission books.[15] Unfortunately there are only few administrative files of the hospital itself. Here we can only draw on the admission books of the hospital[16] and the collection of the Bavarian State Ministry for Education and Culture in the Main State Archive in Munich. There are unfortunately very few administrative records and these only describe the structural processes in the hospital that had to be coordinated with the ministry.[17] For this paper I analysed a sample size of approximately 800 patient records from the period between 1936–1944. A large portion of the patients admitted to the Hospital of Psychiatric and Mental Disorders were men who needed to be checked for their eligibility to receive benefits because of an accident or a disability.[18] The files of patients with psychiatric diagnoses reveal that the most common therapy for restless schizophrenic patients was a "sleep therapy" with Trional, and at times in combination with Veronal. In the sample only four files listed insulin shock therapy (from 1936) as a therapy for schizophrenics, 13 received metrazol shock therapy (from 1937), and 15 were treated with electroconvulsive treatment (from 1940). In the last group two of the patients had been diagnosed with depression. 21 patients were treated with the sleep therapy with Trional and for very restless patients the well-established hydrotherapy with prolonged baths was used.

---

15   UAWü: Patient records of the University Psychiatric Hospital Würzburg.

16   The handwritten data of the admission books that had been organised according to gender have been fully transcribed for the period between 1925–1944 into an excel database for both men and women.

17   HStA M: MK 72463: Chair for Psychiatry and Neurology 1925–1969; MK 72539: University of Würzburg Psychiatric Hospital: Director and medical professionals 1921–1948; MK 72541: University of Würzburg Psychiatric Hospital: Administrative staff, servant position, nursing staff, nurses, 1890–1948; MK 72543: Gebäude der Nervenklinik Würzburg, u. a. Klinikneubau: 1939–1955 (Building of the psychiatric hospital Würzburg, including new construction of the hospital: 1939–1955).

18   Only 33 % of the 1604 men who had been admitted in 1937 were diagnosed with a psychiatric disorder. In 1937 a total of 395 women had been admitted, i. e. a quarter of the male patients. 51 % of the women were diagnosed with psychiatric disorder. Thank you to Andrea Müller for this data collection.

Prolonged narcotic therapy or "sleep therapy"

Prior to the shock therapies in Würzburg the sleep therapy was the preferred treatment choice for schizophrenic patients who were restless and distracted and bothered both other patients and the staff with their uncontrolled loud speaking or screaming. The "sleep therapy" had been introduced in 1920 by the Swiss psychiatrist Jacob Klaesi (1883–1980) as a therapy for schizophrenic patients. After some trials with the barbiturates sulfonmethane and Trional Klaesi used Somnifen to put psychotic patients into a deep sleep for two weeks. His goal was "to gain afterwards in the phase of awakening and affective loosening a psychotherapeutic contact"[19] to the patients who had been hardly accessible at all before. In contrast to the analyses by Schott and Tölle[20] sleep therapy was not a singular experiment by Klaesi. Rather this treatment method was also employed by the psychiatrists Max Müller (1894–1980) in Bern and H. Oberholzer at the Burghölzli asylum in Zurich as a therapy for schizophrenic patients.[21] Pamela Michael has shown how prolonged sleep therapy became an established method for schizophrenic patients in the United Kingdom in the years between the two world wars. She emphasises that prolonged sleep therapy was retained as an alternative even after the introduction of shock therapies for schizophrenics.[22]

The patient records in Würzburg reveal that extremely restless schizophrenic patients were prescribed sleep therapy with Trional and at times also in combination with Veronal. Occasionally this therapy was also used in combination with shock therapies if the patients did not become calmer after multiple shocks and seizures. When the barbiturates were ineffective, the prolonged bath was additionally used – a treatment that had been effective for calming down patients since the 19th century. The sleep that lasted for days on end meant that the nurses had to feed the patients with a tube and wash them. Furthermore the nurses had to monitor and evaluate the patients' state of consciousness and the vital signs because this form of therapy could become quite dangerous for the patients. Often it was impossible, however, to put the patients to sleep despite high doses of Trional. Apparently in Würzburg the doctors shied away from using the stronger barbiturate Somnifen to start a kind of permanent anaesthesia as this was associated with high risks. At the Burghölzli in Zurich the therapy had to be stopped in six of 28 patients due to life-threatening complications. Two patients finally died.[23]

---

19   Schott/Tölle (2006), p. 484.
20   Cf. Schott/Tölle (2006), p. 484.
21   Cf. Windholz/Witherspoon (1993), pp. 88–91.
22   Cf. Michael (2013).
23   Cf. Windholz/Witherspoon (1993), pp. 88.

Convulsion therapy with metrazol and electric shock

Already in 1937 the new shock therapy with metrazol was used in Würzburg
to treat schizophrenic patients. Patients received up to 20 injections metrazol
that resulted in eleptiform convulsions. In the file of patient Rosa Müller[24] we
read that there were three days of "rest" between the individual, at times generalised (that is big eleptiform) seizures. Meduna suggested in his publication
to tie the patient with linen sheets immediately after the injections. This measure, however, proved dangerous for the patients because securing the limbs to
the bed led to bone fractures when the patient was jerking heavily back and
forth.[25] For that reason Anton von Braunmühl suggested to position the patients in a special way: A wedge pillow was to be placed under the knee or the
patient put into an embryo position – on the side with his arms crossed above
the chest and the knees pulled up. To avoid fractures it was important to avoid
convulsions that were too strong and the dose of metrazol had to be "felt out,"
according to Braunmühl.[26] Similarly, Walter Horn, senior physician at the
asylum and nursing home in Werneck,[27] emphasised that "incidents of surgical nature" could be avoided by sparing the patient any type of mechanical
restriction during a convulsion. He continued that a "waist belt" and "foot
straps" were also superfluous "if one put a nurse or carer beside the bed of the
patient when a convulsion is triggered with the order to prevent spasms that
could result in self-harming".[28] In the 13 psychiatric patient files that I analysed for this article, no bone fractures were noted in the patients in Würzburg
who received metrazol therapy.

Horn's description is not the only one that points to the complex tasks the
nurses had to master during the convulsive therapies. The convulsions did not
begin immediately after the injections as the lag time varied between half an
hour and three hours.[29] For that reason the doctors did not have the time to
observe the seizures themselves. The nurses had the important task to intensively observe the patients and monitor their breathing. Furthermore they had
to thoroughly document the progression of the fit and any abnormalities.

---

24 The name of the female patient was pseudonymised, cf. UAWü: Patient records at the
    Neurological Hospital of the University Hospital Würzburg, seq.no. 233/1936 admitted
    on 28/07/1936 and released on 01/07/1937.
25 Bone fractures were also the most common complication during the electroconvulsive
    treatment that was used in Würzburg for the first time in 1940. The literature on the
    history of electroconvulsive treatment does not clearly reveal the precise point in time
    when electroconvulsive treatment with muscle relaxants and anaesthesia began. Cf.
    Heintz (2004); Shorter/Healy (2007).
26 Braunmühl (1942). On the frequency of spinal injuries as a result of convulsive therapies
    see also Schmieder (1942).
27 Until 1940 the sanatorium and nursing home Werneck was one of the two institutions to
    which chronically psychiatric patients were transferred from the Psychiatric Department
    of the University Hospital Würzburg. In 1940 the patients from Werneck were trans-
    ferred to the sanatorium in Lohr or directly to a killing centre.
28 Horn (1939), p. 230.
29 Cf. Meduna (1937), p. 13.

Meduna underlines in his book how much the doctors depended on well-trained nurses.

> Since the effect of the camphor injection was completely unreliable the patients who were chosen to receive treatment had to be accommodated in a special room and a trained nurse had to be at all times with the patients. The latter fact is particularly important because the camphor injection often does not cause convulsions but a delirium that is a side effect of psychomotor restlessness.[30]

Nurses had to be able to act correctly in a case of emergency. In contrast to the files on insulin shock therapy there is no documentation written by nurses on patients on metrazol shock therapy. The doctors' notes contain nonetheless detailed descriptions of the convulsions that are most probably based on the nurses' observations. For instance we read in the file of the previously mentioned patient Rosa Müller: "typical convulsion with increased pallor, without wetting herself, duration 47" [minutes, K.N.]. Or, four days later:

> After 18" pat. becomes very red, is shaking, duration of this state 90". No typical convulsion. During this exceptional state, she did not speak a word and was lying completely calmly in bed. Afterwards she was very tranquil, complained about pain at the injection site in her arm and asked for a compress.[31]

The last description illustrates how long such episodes could last. The doctors would hardly have had the time to sit at a patient's bed for nearly two hours and to watch her. These observations were therefore most likely written by a nurse who took on this important task for a doctor. The behaviour and thus the mental state of a patient was mainly monitored by the nurses on the wards. After eleven "metrazol injections" Rosa Müller's behaviour is described in the doctor's notes as follows:

> Unchanged situation. Pat. still often screams loudly […] Does not recognise people. Becomes aggressive. Very irritable. Bad intake of food, often spills her meals. Needs sedatives. Lately maintains her very reduced body weight. Keeps herself clean. Often sits in bed in completely odd positions, pushing her head into her hands or the pillow and scratching her face because she grinds her finger nails into the flesh. When her relatives visited she assaulted them, screamed loudly, slapped the sister and ripped buttons off her attire. Always very negative. Emotional outbursts beyond measure.

While doctors also gained an impression of the state of the patients when they made their rounds, the detailed observations were the nurses' contributions, meaning that they provided the essential basis for the encompassing evaluation of the patients. The files of those patients who had previously undergone a metrazol shock therapy strikingly document how the patients fought against the new injections. After she woke from her unconsciousness Luise Huber[32] for example screamed "wildly for help, insulted the doctors and nurses, called

---

30 Cf. Meduna (1937), p. 9.
31 Cf. UAWü: Patient records at the Neurological Hospital of the University Hospital Würzburg, seq.no. 233/1936 admitted on 28/07/1936 and released on 01/07/1937.
32 The name of the female patient was pseudonymised, cf. UAWü: Patient records at the University Psychiatric Hospital Würzburg, seq.no. 75/1940 admitted on 22/03/1940 and released on 30/060/1940.

them murderers and pushed hard to get out of bed". Her resolute resistance against the torturous therapy earned her the addition of "primitive personality" to her diagnosis of schizophrenia.[33]

The files of the patients who underwent electroconvulsive treatment at the Hospital of Psychiatric and Mental Disorders in Würzburg from 1940 also reveal severe resistance against this therapy. The patient Anna Müller[34] had to be held by three nurses on the first day of the convulsion therapy because she fought using her entire body strength and screamed at the same time with all her might. Three days later they needed already four nurses to hold the patient in check who was "most forcefully" fighting. Finally the therapy had to be terminated due to the "strong resistance" of the patient. Three weeks later a new attempt was made and the patient no longer fought against it. The treatment did not however show any effect. She was admitted and released for another three times and each time electroconvulsive treatment was used – each time without success.[35] In the patient records of the schizophrenics treated with electroconvulsive treatment the nurses emerge merely as disciplining agents. The nurses' close observations only indirectly surface in the comprehensive descriptions of the patients' behaviour in the everyday life at the ward that are contained in the patient history.

Next I address the records on insulin shock therapy since these sources directly present the nurses as agents.

Insulin shock therapy and documentation

Before Sakel treated schizophrenic patients with insulin he had observed in his treatment of morphine addicts that their psychological well-being significantly improved after they received insulin. In Würzburg patients suffering from morphinism were also treated with insulin.[36] Sakel divided the insulin shock therapy into four parts: 1. The "initiation phase" during which increasing doses of insulin were administered; 2. The "shock phase" that was characterised through the hypoglycaemic shock; 3. The phase with resting days, and 4. The phase with smaller doses of insulin and an early disruption of hypoglycaemia. Especially in the first phase the patients needed to be monitored very carefully. For cardiovascular management pulse and blood pressure had to be frequently measured and documented. Furthermore one side effect of hypoglycaemia is hunger that the nurses had to pay special attention to. Based on

---

33   Cf. UAWü: Patient records at the University Psychiatric Hospital Würzburg, 1940, seq. no. 293 admitted on 22/08/1943 and released on 02/09/1943.

34   The name of the patient was pseudonymised, cf. UAWü: Patient records at the Neurological Hospital of the University Hospital Würzburg, seq.no. 75/1940 admitted on 22/3/1940 and released on 30/6/1940.

35   Cf. UAWü: Patient records at the University Psychiatric Hospital Würzburg, 1940, seq. no. 75/1940 admitted on 22/3/1940 and released on 30/6/1940.

36   Cf. UAWü: Patient records, University Neurological Hospital Würzburg: seq.no. 16/1937: here a doctor who was a morphine addict was treated with insulin.

his experiences with the therapy the senior physician at the Eglfing-Haar asylum, Anton von Braunmühl, recommended in his manual to interrupt the hypoglycaemia after the third insulin hour if a "hunger agitation" occurred.[37] With this advice he deviated from Sakel's method. This book was also available at the library of the Hospital of Psychiatric and Mental Disorders in Würzburg.

The second phase, the "shock phase" was the most critical one. Hence Braunmühl recommended keeping a shock board for each patient.

> Like any other observations (such as time of sleepiness, seizures, spasms, time and method of waking the patient) the nurses copied in the data from the board into their own daily chart. During the shock phase the nursing staff continuously keeps an eye on the patient. They measure pulse and breathing, watch the colour of the face etc. Comatose patients are to be positioned according to Sakel's recommendation with cushions in an elevated position and the head turned to the side so that it rests below the shoulder. This prevents the saliva of heavily salivating patients from passing into the airways.[38]

These depictions illustrate how crucial the cautious actions and knowledge of the nursing staff was for the event free completion of this dangerous therapy. Nurses also had to be able to evaluate whether a patient was in a "half shock" or a complete "shock". In the former the patient would still respond to painful stimuli but could no longer drink anything, a complete shock had been reached when the patient no longer responded to any stimuli, which the nurses were supposed to test by strongly pinching. Accordingly, Braunmühl recommended sorting the "staff question" when setting up an insulin ward: "For nursing staff we calculate one nurse for six patients for the first two insulin hours."[39] An additional nurse and a doctor were supposed to be available on call. "We cannot warn enough against positioning insufficient numbers of staff. The nurses who are chosen and examined due to their special achievement and reliability are allowed to perform the intramuscular insulin injections."[40]

How the staff issue was organised in the hospital in Würzburg we can only indirectly deduct from the sources. In 1937 the Psychiatric and Neurological Hospital housed 120 patients.[41] The patients were looked after by a total of 22 nurses from the Catholic congregation of the Daughters of the Holiest Redeemer ("Kongregation der Töchter des allerheiligsten Erlösers"), i.e. the

---

37   Braunmühl (1938), p. 18.
38   Braunmühl (1938), pp. 26–27.
39   Braunmühl (1938), p. 2.
40   Braunmühl (1938), p. 2.
41   The director was Martin Reichardt whose areas of expertise were brain research and the evaluation of accidents. Until 1939 the senior physician was Werner Heyde who subsequently took on Reichardt's teaching position after he had become an emeritus. At the same time there were five male and one female assistant doctors (comparable to today's registrars) who worked at the hospital: Wilhelm Schumacher; Richard Krämer, Karl Stössel, Hans Klaassen, Wolfgang Steinkopff, and Elisabeth Pawlik, cf. Laehr (1937), p. 114.

so called "redeemer sisters"[42] and seven male nurses.[43] The ongoing requests that the director of the hospital, Martin Reichardt, sent to the Bavarian State Ministry for Education and Culture in the 1930s speaks for a permanent lack of nursing staff.[44] The few male nurses were apparently not highly educated as their applications for pay raises that they sent to the ministry illustrate. The letters are full of spelling errors, and they even had trouble writing the name of the hospital correctly as in one letter it is named each time as "Psysiatric Hospital" (Psysiatrische Klinik).[45] If we assume that presumably the nurse who could write the best wrote the letters to the ministry, the letters allow conclusions on the educational level the male nurses in Würzburg had achieved. Thus it seems very likely that the task of complex monitoring, the control of vital signs and the documentation for the insulin patients were rather entrusted to the denominational (female) nurses.

Documentation of nursing in Würzburg

One of the first three schizophrenic patients who were treated in Würzburg with the new Sakel therapy was the 25-year-old servant Otto Oberhuber.[46] He was taken to the Psychiatric and Neurological Hospital at the University of Würzburg because he was "restless" and talked "nonsensically". His diagnosis at admission was "dementia praecox" which was changed later in the hospital to the more modern clinical diagnose "schizophrenia". It was here that the staff also observed that the servant sounded like a "lunatic" and wrote down verbatim what he had said. The doctors responded to his first "agitated attack" with morphine-scopaline injections. The graph in his file reveals that he did not only daily receive injections with sedatives during the first days of his stay but also continuously while he was under insulin coma therapy.[47] The graphs do not contain the administrations of insulin and a documentation of "shocks" versus "half-shocks" is equally missing. The insulin shock therapy is mentioned on a report that was later inserted, which covers about two thirds of an A4 sheet of paper and had been written on a typewriter. This documentation appears improvised and indicates that this was one of the first healing

---

42 Cf. also the Archive of the congregation of the daughters of the Holiest redeemer, file on the University Psychiatric Hospital Würzburg. The "redeemer sisters" began working at the University Psychiatric Hospital in 1897, initially with seven nurses. They ended their assignment here in 1952 mainly due to a lack of new recruits in the congregation.

43 Cf. Laehr (1937), p. 114.

44 Cf. HStA M: MK 72541: University of Würzburg Psychiatric Hospital, administrative staff, servant positions, nursing staff, nurses, 1890–1948.

45 HStA M: MK 72541, Letter from 11 August 1932.

46 The name of the patient was pseudonymised. UAWü: Patient records at the University Psychiatric Hospital, seq.no. 1/1936 admitted on 01/01/1936 and released on 04/04/1936.

47 UAWü: Patient records at the University Psychiatric Hospital, seq.no. 1/1936 admitted on 01/01/1936 and released on 04/04/1936.

attempts using the insulin shock therapy in Würzburg. Indeed, in contrast to previous assumptions by other authors[48] Würzburg was one of the first hospitals that used Sakel's therapy in the German Reich, after Wilhelm Ederle (1901–1966) had begun already in 1935 with therapy attempts at the Hospital of Psychiatric and Mental Disorders at the University of Gießen. It took another three years until Anton von Braunmühl published his manual on the "Insulinschockbehandlung der Schizophrenie" (Insulin Shock Therapy of Schizophrenia) that contained his detailed instructions on both administering the therapy and documenting it.[49] Braunmühl's manual made it very clear that observation, measurements and documentation were tasks for the nursing staff. His description reveals how crucial the nurses' thorough work of observing and documenting was for the doctors' decision making in the course of the treatment.[50] Precise instructions for nurses on how to act during an insulin shock therapy can only be found in a textbook for nurses from the time after the Second World War. This book was published when nursing in psychiatry had become a fixed part of the nursing training in West Germany.[51] The three phases of insulin shock therapy are explained in detail in this textbook: 1 initiation phase; 2 shock phase, and 3 post-treatment phase. Here we can also read how the "half shock" could be distinguished from a "full shock" and that the former had to be entered into the chart as a semi-circle and the latter as a whole circle. The nurses were advised that the patients not only needed intensive monitoring and focus during the first two phases but also in the third phase, and then particularly at night, because the endogenous increased insulin release in response to the treatment could lead to another hypoglycaemic shock.[52] We might assume, however, that the nurses who were chosen to participate in insulin shock therapy received special training at the hospital or asylum respectively. Unfortunately in Würzburg no materials have survived that allow conclusions as to when the nurses received such instructions and what the particular content was.

The development of how insulin shock therapy was documented also emerges from the patient records. In the early patient records from 1936 the chart contains pulse and temperature in the same way as it was documented before the introduction of insulin shock therapy. Notes on the patients' behav-

---

48 In contrast to the history of the introduction of insulin shock therapy in the German Reich provided by Hammann-Roth, the psychiatrists in Würzburg began in February 1936 at the latest to use the new shock therapy. Cf. Hammann-Roth (2001), p. 54: The author refers to a headline in the Psychiatrisch-Neurologischen Wochenschrift, cf. "Übersicht über die nach der Methode der Wiener Psychiatrischen Klinik (Hypoglykämie-Chok) behandelten Schizophreniefälle", in: Psychiatrisch-Neurologische Wochenschrift 35 (1936), p. 423. The reference is the patient record, UAWü: Patient records at the University Psychiatric Hospital, seq.no. 1/1936, that show that insulin shock therapy was started on 2/2/1936.
49 Braunmühl (1938).
50 Wiedemann (1939).
51 Only in 1957 psychiatric nursing became an obligatory part of the nursing curriculum.
52 Deutsche Schwesternschaft (1958), pp. 675–679.

iour are usually only part of the doctors' notes. Here the junior doctors made relatively schematic entries on the administration of insulin and both the physical and psychological responses. In a patient file from 1940, in addition to the chart with the usual vital signs – pulse, temperature, body weight, and stool – the insulin administration over a period of six weeks was included as a rising curve (40 units up to 122 units insulin). Furthermore the "shocks" are included as blank red circles, the "half-shocks" as blank red semi-circles, and "epileptic seizures" as solid red circles (Figure 1). On separate sheets the insulin units, the state of consciousness, the patient's behaviour, the various "shocks", epileptic convulsions, the patient's ability to drink, which is an indicator for the patient's state of consciousness, and the use of a feeding tube were documented. Furthermore the file contains a fever chart and the exact documentation of fluid intake. This comprehensive documentation of the progress of the therapy illustrates not only the huge effort nurses put into the written documentation but also how thorough and carefully they monitored the patients. In another patient record from 1941 another step for systematising the documentation of the nurses' intensive monitoring of patients during insulin shock therapy becomes apparent: Now all the values were entered into a form with dedicated fields: pulse, temperature, intake of fluids, weight, and stool on the one hand and insulin units, the various "shocks", their depth (with the usual circles) and their duration (with a vertical red dotted line along the time scale) as well as T for "Trinken" (drink) and S for "Sonde" (feeding tube) on the other hand (Figure 2). The psychiatrist at the asylum Osnabrück had developed a similar special chart form for the combined insulin and metrazol shock therapy already in 1939 because he wanted to "train" the nurses in more thorough monitoring. Apparently the nursing staff was very happy about the new form as they were now spared the inconvenience of filling in multiple documents. For the doctors the advantage was that they could see all observations and measurements at once in a glance.[53] On the back of the form the behaviour was supposed to be entered in a table: "under hypoglycaemia" and "out of hypoglycaemia". The nurses' notes are much more detailed in these columns than previously on the extra sheet without a provided structure. In the following section we will analyse the nurses' descriptions of the patients' behaviour in more detail. What is the connection to the doctor's notes, which observations did the doctors make, are there additional descriptions of the patients' behaviour that can only stem from the nurses but are not part of the notes on the sheet for insulin therapy?

Reconstructions of nursing practice

The thorough, time-intensive observation and the qualified actions of the nurses were essential to the successful treatment with the new shock therapies. The sources do not reveal how the intensive observation during insulin coma

---

53   Wiedemann (1939).

therapy and the close monitoring and documentation of pulse, temperature, and blood sugar was organised in which would have been a considerable feat given the severe shortage of staff. The nursing practice as it is documented in the patient records illustrates, however, how carefully the nurses performed and recorded the monitoring and measurements of the patients. In addition they were apparently capable of responding to critical life-threatening situations by administering glucose solutions or by using a feeding tube that they had previously put in place. In addition to the handwritten notes on the form for insulin shock therapy there are more detailed descriptions of the patients' behaviour from the daily life at the ward. These appear in reports that the doctors had typed but that were clearly informed by the reports the nurses had provided. Given the staff shortage at the University Hospital in Würzburg we might assume that the time-intensive work of closely observing and often repeatedly measuring all parameters for the insulin coma therapy were conducted at the expense of the remaining patients. Among the 800 patient records that I worked through there are very few files that describe this particular somatic therapy that was very popular elsewhere. Yet the administrative files reveal that in 1941 one female doctor was in charge of conducting insulin treatments.[54] This is an indication that at least during the 1940s a larger number of insulin shock therapies were being conducted.[55]

Using a concrete case example I will now illustrate the specific nursing practices used in insulin coma therapy: In October 1941 the twenty year old Katharina Maier[56] was admitted with a diagnosis of schizophrenia and catatonic stupor (rigidity of the whole body). The patient file by the doctor's hand contains the following description of her behaviour:

> Lies completely impassively in bed, at times she gets up and walks aimlessly through the room. Hardly any spontaneous utterances and if so, then only incomprehensible word bites. Does not answer to questions but vacantly looks at the doctor without any interest.[57]

To prevent the patient from walking around aimlessly she was "tied". Furthermore it was noted that she "caused quite some trouble with eating."[58]

---

54 HStA M, MK 72539: University of Würzburg Psychiatric Hospital: Director and medical professionals 1921–1948, Letter to the ministry by Senior Physician of the Würzburg Hospital, Dr. Karl Stößel representing Director Professor Dr. Werner Heyde, on 01/06/1940.

55 This impression is hardened by the fact that I had to search through fewer boxes with patient records from 1940 and 1941 to find files with insulin shock therapy than in the early years. I had to go through a significantly higher number of boxes to find a file from the early phase of insulin shock therapy in Würzburg. Indeed there were only three cases in 1936.

56 The name of the patient was pseudonymised. UAWü: Patient records at the University Psychiatric Hospital, seq.no. 314/1941 admitted on 13/10/1941 and released on 03/12/1941.

57 Cf. UAWü: Patient records at the University Psychiatric Hospital, seq.no. 314/1941 admitted on 13/10/1941 and released on 03/12/1941.

58 Cf. UAWü: Patient records at the University Psychiatric Hospital, seq.no. 314/1941 admitted on 13/10/1941 and released on 03/12/1941.

One week after her admission the doctors started her on an "insulin treatment." Her father had given his consent in writing with merely one sentence –
it is not apparent from the file to what extent he had really been informed
about the dangers of the therapy. On the back of the chart the nurses noted
the behaviour under hypoglycaemia on the second day of the therapy:
"mainly restless", and out of hypoglycaemia: "The pat[ient] repeatedly cries
and is at times violent. P[atient] had a visitor whom she did not recognise." A
few days later, the nurses noted a reaction to an "electroconvulsive treatment"
that the patient additionally received to bring her out of her catatonic stupor:
"Afterwards very agitated, screamed, talked to her environment that she could
not bear it due to the pain. Received inj[ections] of m[orphine] s[copaline].
Pat[ient] said that she wanted to lie down beneath [sic] the train tracks." The
doctor copied this handwritten note by the nurses verbatim in his typed report, including the wrong preposition "beneath" ("unter"). On the following
day the insulin coma therapy was continued. Since the patient was "very agitated" and "wildly" screamed in "bed" when she was hypoglycaemic she was
brought out of the state of shock. On the following day the nurses noted that
the patient had recognised her visitors, got out of bed for the first time and
behaved "fairly calmly."[59]

In between the patient received a new "electroconvulsive treatment" that
resulted in strong back pain and had apparently also affected her lower inci-
sors that had become loose. A few days later the nurses registered that the
patient was "quite balanced in herself." In the doctor's report we read in more
detail:

> She gets up […] in the afternoon, makes her bed herself and sits down calmly in the
> common room. She does not engage in any activity yet and does not spontaneously talk
> to others. The nurse always asks her to go into the garden with her. When doing so she
> behaves very well and does not run away. She eats by herself and drinks a lot. She asked
> where she is and how long she's been here.[60]

Her "balanced" and "calm" behaviour continued also in the fifth week of insulin coma therapy. However, it was still regarded as a sign of the disease that the
patient did not want to discuss her disease. During the sixth week of therapy,
she underwent two additional electroshocks. The medical report states that
the patient "believably" denies "any psychotic experiences." Since she still
refused to discuss her disease, she could only be released from the hospital
against the doctor's advice. A letter the patient wrote to the director of the
hospital in 1956 implies that she never had any other psychotic phases or
other disease symptoms after her treatment. Even contemporaries could not
have clearly decided whether this long lasting remission was a spontaneous
remission or a result of the therapy. The Würzburg psychiatrist Rudolf Tangermann noticed that the proportion of spontaneous remissions in schizophren-

59   Cf. UAWü: Patient records at the University Psychiatric Hospital, seq.no. 314/1941 ad-
     mitted on 13/10/1941 and released on 03/12/1941.
60   UAWü: Patient records at the University Psychiatric Hospital, seq.no. 314/1941 admitted
     on 13/10/1941 and released on 03/12/1941.

ics who did not receive shock therapy in the Werneck asylum hardly differed from the remission rate discussed in the publication on insulin shock therapies. He assumed that the mentioned cases of remission after insulin shock therapy could just as well have been spontaneous remissions.[61]

Finally we note that this case study reveals that not only the nurses' thorough monitoring of the patient's measurements was decisive for the evaluation of the course of the therapy. Rather the comments regarding significant changes in the patient's behaviour were important for the carers to note signs of her improvement.

For other patients the insulin coma therapy was not as "trouble free" and "successful". Thus in 1940 the 32 year old Ottilie Schmitt[62] was transferred as unhealed to the recovery and nursing asylum Lohr after 13 weeks of insulin coma therapy during which the patient nearly died in a generalised seizure, caused by an additional generalised seizure during electroconvulsive treatment. To calm her down the nurses went back to hydrotherapy. Nurses used a prolonged bath in hot water already towards the end of the 19th century to calm down or discipline extremely restless patients. Similarly, in the 38 year old Marie Obermaier[63] who had been diagnosed with schizophrenia, daily prolonged baths proved apparently more effective than the shock therapy with insulin that had been tested on her for weeks. She was also transferred to Lohr as "unhealed" for permanent care.

Conclusion

For the implementation, monitoring, and final evaluation of the success of the therapies that had been introduced in the 1930s and 1940s well trained, thorough, and cautiously acting nursing staff was vital. Manfred Sakel and Ladislaus Meduna, the inventors of insulin shock therapy and metrazol shock therapy, shared this insight already in their first publications. It is remarkable that nurses only left traces in the sources only in the context of these therapies that required a good understanding of technology. While the routine patient observations that they conducted daily on the wards were written down for the psychiatrists, they were not deemed worthy for keeping after the doctors had copied the most important aspects into the patient records. The reports on the daily nursing routine were not filed in the records like the nurses' reports on insulin shock therapy. This suggests a hierarchy between "normal" psychiatric care and the specialised care for the shock therapies.

61 Cf. the controversy between Rudolf Tangermann from Würzburg (!) and Moritz Schnidtmann from the asylum Eglfing-Haar; Tangermann (1942); Schnidtmann (1943).
62 The name of the patient was pseudonymised. UAWü: Patient records at the University Psychiatric Hospital, seq.no. 329/1941 admitted on 28/10/1941 and released on 01/11/1941.
63 The name of the patient was pseudonymised. UAWü: Patient records at the University Psychiatric Hospital, seq.no. 329/1940 admitted on 14/12/1940 and released on 28/05/1941.

Nurses who could confidently handle these therapies that were very dangerous for the patients became irreplaceable in their respective hospital or asylum. Yet, this clear specialisation within the profession of psychiatric nurse did not lead to a valorisation of it.

The patients presumably identified the nurses with the torturous and – due to the violence – degrading therapies because they bore the major burden of the work when conducting the shock therapies. It was them who used force when holding the patients who fought against the metrazol injection or the attachment of the electrodes for the electroconvulsive treatment.

How nurses of shock therapies were perceived by the public can be nicely seen in a film presentation and the responses it received from the public. In the 1948 American movie "The Snake Pit," psychiatric nurses were presented as decisive promoters and unmerciful executors of electroconvulsive treatment. The film was shown in Germany in 1950 under the title "Die Schlangengrube." While the majority of the German critics evaluated the presentation of the situation in the asylum as particularly close to reality, the "experts" vehemently protested against the negative depiction of the "shock treatment". The psychiatrists who joined the discussion protected the nurses who had been presented in the film as "too militaristic". The head physician of a "spa asylum" even demanded: "This film needs to be forbidden!" as it would undermine the "trust in the psychiatrist."[64] In 1954 the Würzburg daily newspaper "Mainpost" published an article titled "An der Füchsleinstraße[65] gibt es keine "Schlangengrube"" (In English "In the Füchsleinstraße there is no snake pit"). The article presents to the public the new university psychiatric hospital renovated in a modern style: "And even while we had not expected a "Snake Pit" in the manner of the world famous novel and film that came out a few years ago, we were quite astonished by the friendly atmosphere in the whole house."[66] The term "Snake Pit" was an indirect reference to the shock therapies feared by the public that had become a symbol of the inhumane psychiatric treatments.

How the nurses themselves regarded the shock therapies and how they evaluated their own contribution has unfortunately not been recorded.

---

64   Cf. ""Giftspritzen" gegen "Schlangenbiss"". Berliner Morgenecho from 12/6/1950. In the Spandauer Volksblatt "experts" also shared their concern about the film, cf. "Fachleute über "Die Schlangengrube"", In: Spandauer Volksblatt from 10/6/1950. District doctors who were responsible to "transfer mentally ill" patients to the asylum recommended to show the film only to "doctors, nurses and carers" in private performances particularly because of the scene with the electroconvulsive treatment. The newspaper articles are from the press archive at the Academy of Film and Television in Potsdam.

65   Füchsleinstraße was the address of the University Psychiatric Hospital. A typical saying had always been: "You will end up in Füchsleinstraße!" After the hospital had been renamed in 2014 into "Centre for psychological health" the address has now also recently changed. The square in front of the hospital was named after a former patient who became a victim of the Action T4: Margarete-Höppel-Platz.

66   Mainpost/148, Thursday, 1 July 1954, p. 3.

Bibliography

Archival sources

Archive of the congregation of the daughters of the Holiest redeemer (Archiv der Kongregation der Töchter des allerheiligsten Erlösers)

Record on the University Psychiatric Hospital Würzburg.

Bayerisches Hauptstaatsarchiv München (HStA M):

MK 72541: Universität Würzburg Psychiatrische Klinik, Verwaltungspersonal, Diener-Stellen, Pflegepersonal, Schwestern, 1890–1948. (University of Würzburg Psychiatric Hospital, administrative staff, servant positions, nursing staff, nurses, 1890–1948.)
MK 72463: Ordentlicher Lehrstuhl für Psychiatrie und Neurologie 1925–1969 (Chair for Psychiatry and Neurology 1925–1969)
MK 72539: University of Würzburg Psychiatric Hospital: Direktor und ärztliches Personal 1921–1948. (Director and medical professionals 1921–1948.)
MK 72543: Gebäude der Nervenklinik Würzburg, u. a. Klinikneubau: 1939–1955 (Building of the psychiatric hospital Würzburg, including new construction of the hospital: 1939–1955).

University Archive Würzburg (UAWü)

Patient records of the University Psychiatric Hospital Würzburg.

Press archive of the Academy of Film and Television in Potsdam:

O. A.: "'Giftspritzen' gegen 'Schlangenbiss'". In: Berliner Morgenecho from 12/6/1950.
O. A.: "Fachleute über 'Die Schlangengrube'", In: Spandauer Volksblatt from 10/6/1950.

Printed sources

Braunmühl, Anton v.: Die Insulinschockbehandlung der Schizophrenie (unter Berücksichtigung des Cardiazolkrampfes). Ein Leitfaden für die Praxis. Berlin 1938.
Braunmühl, Anton v.: Aus der Praxis der Krampftherapie. Lagerung der Krampfenden. Optimale Krampfschwelle. In: Allgemeine Zeitschrift für Psychiatrie und psychisch-gerichtliche Medizin 120 (1942), pp. 147–157.
Deutsche Schwesternschaft e. V. (ed.): Die Pflege des kranken Menschen. Lehrbuch für Krankenpflegeschulen, Stuttgart 1958.
Horn, Walter: Zwischenfälle chirurgischer Art bei der Krampf- und Schocktherapie. In: Psychiatrisch-Neurologische Wochenschrift 41 (1939), 19, pp. 229–231.
Laehr, Heinrich: Verzeichnis der Anstalten in alphabetischer Reihenfolge. In: Allgemeine Zeitschrift für Psychiatrie und psychisch-gerichtliche Medizin 106 (1937), pp. 1–164.
Meduna, Ladislaus: Die Konvulsionstherapie der Schizophrenie. Halle a. S. 1937.
Morgenthaler, Walter: Pflege der Gemüts- und Geisteskranken. Bern; Berlin 1930.
Oberholzer, W.: Arbeiten zur Insulinschocktherapie der Schizophrenie. In: Allgemeine Zeitschrift für Psychiatrie und ihre Grenzgebiete 114 (1940), pp. 271–287.

Sakel, Manfred: Neue Behandlungsmethode der Schizophrenie. Wien; Leipzig 1935.
Schmieder, Fritz: Zur Häufigkeit und Bedeutung der Wirbelsäulenschädigung bei Krampf- und Schockverfahren. In: Allgemeine Zeitschrift für Psychiatrie und psychisch-gerichtliche Medizin 121 (1942), pp. 141–180.
Schnidtmann, Moritz: Spontan-Remissionen bei Schizophrenie. In: Allgemeine Zeitschrift für Psychiatrie und psychisch-gerichtliche Medizin 122 (1943), pp. 87–93.
Tangermann, Rudolf: Spontan-Remissionen bei Schizophrenie. In: Allgemeine Zeitschrift für Psychiatrie und psychisch-gerichtliche Medizin 121 (1942), pp. 36–57.
Thumm, M.: Über den Stand der Insulin- und Cardiazolbehandlung. Literaturbericht. In: Allgemeine Zeitschrift für Psychiatrie und ihre Grenzgebiete 109 (1938), pp. 280–325.
Übersicht über die nach der Methode der Wiener Psychiatrischen Klinik (Hypoglykämie-Chok) behandelten Schizophreniefälle. In: Psychiatrisch-Neurologische Wochenschrift 35 (1936), p. 423.
Wiedemann, Fritz: Einführung einer Kurve für die Insulinschock- und Cardiazolkrampftherapie. In: Psychiatrisch-Neurologische Wochenschrift 41 (1939), 48, pp. 495–499.

Secondary research literature

Beyer, Christof: Die Einführung der "heroischen" Therapien in den Heil- und Pflegeanstalten der Provinz Hannover 1936–1939 In: Schmuhl, Hans-Walter; Roelcke, Volker (ed.): "Heroische Therapien" Die deutsche Psychiatrie im internationalen Vergleich 1918–1945, Wallstein: Göttingen 2013, pp. 233–267.
Braunschweig, Sabine: Zwischen Aufsicht und Betreuung. Berufsbildung und Arbeitsalltag der Psychiatriepflege am Beispiel der Basler Heil- und Pflegeanstalt Friedmatt, 1886–1960. Zürich 2013.
Hamann-Roth, Matthias: Die Einführung der Insulinschocktherapie im Deutschen Reich 1935 bis 1937. Wetzlar 2001.
Heintz, Erik Robert: Die Einführung der Elektrokrampftherapie an der Psychiatrischen und Nervenklinik der Universität München 1941 bis 1945. Diss. Med. 2004.
Michael, Pamela: Prolonged Narcosis Therapy during the Inter-War Years. In: Schmuhl, Hans-Walter; Roelcke, Volker (ed.): "Heroische Therapien" Die deutsche Psychiatrie im internationalen Vergleich 1918–1945, Göttingen 2013, pp. 114–130.
Schott, Heinz; Tölle, Rainer: Geschichte der Psychiatrie. Krankheitslehren, Irrwege, Behandlungsformen. München 2006.
Shorter, Edward; Healy, David: Shock Therapy. A History of Electroconvulsive Treatment in Mental Illness. New Jersey 2007.
Windholz, G.; Witherspoon, L.H.: Sleep as a cure for schizophrenia: a historical episode. In: History of Psychiatry 5 (1993), pp. 83–93.

Treating through Threat and Fear – Nurses and the Fever Unit at the Ontario Hospital, Toronto 1940–1951

Thomas Foth / Cheryl McWatters / Jette Lange / Mary B. Connell

Summary

In 1939 the Ontario Hospital, Toronto, initiated a special fever unit for patients with neurosyphilis that was run exclusively by nurses. In this new treatment facility, patients were placed in a high-temperature cabinet in order to elevate their body temperature (105 degrees Fahrenheit up to 8 hours was estimated as the most effective therapeutic approach). According to the advocates of physically induced fever, this form of therapy had decisive advantages over earlier forms of fever treatments. They argued that traditional fever treatments, particularly malarial inoculation, required long hospitalizations for patients, subjected them to the infection of a second disease with consequent debilitation, and were not easily controlled. Furthermore, reactions could become severe enough to endanger patients' lives. Psychiatrists advocated for this new form of fever treatment because patients did not necessarily require hospitalization; they could receive the treatment one day a week and, if necessary, could return to their usual occupation. In addition, persons who had been infected with syphilis but were not yet showing any clinical symptoms could be treated with this therapy as a kind of preventive intervention.

This chapter is based on an in-depth analysis of two medical records from this fever unit and aims to better understand the roles and practices of the nurses running the unit. As the nurses' notes illustrate, the physical fever treatment led to many life-threatening consequences for the patients (e.g. respiratory or cardiac arrest); although psychiatrists called them simply "nurse technicians," nurses working on this ward had to manage highly complex care situations. The notes also highlight that not only did the nurses randomly combine different therapies (i.e. continuous baths, physical restraint, chemical restraint, and Electro-Convulsive Therapy (ECT)), they also applied them in an unsystematic manner. Patients suffered under these "heroic treatments," and were often described as completely helpless and disoriented. The notes also clearly indicate that the success of the "therapies" was based on the nurses' perception of "positive" changes in patients' behaviour," meaning that patients better integrated into the asylum's system of regulation.

The Fever Unit at the Ontario Hospital, Toronto

In 1940, the Ontario Hospital, Toronto (better known as 999 Queen Street) installed a fever unit for the treatment of patients with neuro-syphilis, a late stage of the sexually-transmitted disease syphilis, leading to what was called at that time general paresis. Patients were placed in a high-temperature cabinet filled with moist hot air in order to elevate their body temperature (105 degrees Fahrenheit and up to 8 hours was estimated as the most effective therapeutic approach). Advocates of the fever unit emphasized that this form of treatment was effective and very comfortable for patients. Our chapter aims to understand how these treatments were administered and what the role of nurses in the fever unit was. We highlight that the medical literature of the period reported about multiple life-threatening effects of fever treatments.

While these effects were well known and studied, the many precautionary measures recommended in the literature to minimize them had never been implemented in the Ontario Hospital's fever unit.

The analysis demonstrates that patients suffered incredibly, were systematically led to the edge of death, and regularly experienced respiratory or cardiac arrest. We hypothesize that the continued use of fever treatments went beyond the "biological treatment" of neuro-syphilis; they were also aimed at disciplining patient behaviour. Our argument is supported by the fact that the US Public Health Service had announced (in 1943) that penicillin was active against the syphilis spirochete, a treatment without any of the side effects of the fever treatment.[1] Yet the unit continued well into the 1950s, often combining different shock treatments (i. e. Electro-Convulsive Therapy), different forms of physical restraints (i. e. continuous baths, Cold Water Packs (CWP) and isolation) and sedatives. After 1943, fever treatments were sometimes combined with penicillin.[2]

Furthermore, we contend that nurses played the major role in disciplining patients since the fever unit was run under their sole responsibility. Nurses managed the unit and the treatments ordered for the patients, which were carried out without the presence of psychiatrists. The nursing records in patient charts, our main research focus for this chapter, demonstrate that nurses systematically conducted patients into a "twilight state" between life and death. Even in "emergency" situations, rarely did they ever call in any physicians.

In the next section, we provide an overview of the rationale for the chemical and mechanical treatment and a brief description of the so-called temperature cabinets. We confront Bromley's claims of an unproblematic treatment, which could be carried out by anyone without special training, with what was known at this time about the dangerous implications of this kind of treatment. We further demonstrate that the vast majority of patients never received treatments according to the treatment plan originally introduced by Bromley, due to the massive occurrence of life-threatening incidences. Treatments were rather randomly administered. Using two individual cases of patients treated in the unit, we outline how the treatments were applied and the role which nurses played in the administration of these treatments. We further highlight how these treatments were combined with a multitude of other disciplinary technologies and how these contributed to psychiatric practice. We conclude our study in terms of a more theoretical perspective to foster our understanding of how these treatments were an important means to strengthen psychiatric and nursing power in psychiatric practice.

1   Kruif (1943).
2   Hospitals Division Department of Health (1950).

The medical records used for this analysis

The case records used for our analysis stem from 451 case files that are preserved in four separate boxes at the Archives of Ontario (see reference for details). From the Fever Unit's treatment lists, we assume that these were all cases treated in this unit between 1941 to 1953 as patient data are incomplete for the years 1940 to 1943. Table 1 begins only in 1943 and breakdowns the treatment by gender, year, number and hours of treatment. Although the treatment lists initially depict that more men than women were treated for neuro-syphillis (as was consistent with public health statistics of the time), they no longer differentiate by gender after 1948, and from 1951 on, they are incomplete in general. The unit continued until 1953 even though a sharp decline in patients occurred as soon as 1944, which might be due to the limited success of treatment, despite Bromley's claims, and partly to the introduction of penicillin in 1943. Two types of records for patients treated in the Fever Unit exist – one from the regular ward (the actual medical record) and another kept separately that contained only the fever charts (actually these charts were treatment protocols) and other documents strictly related to the fever treatment. These latter documents were written by nurses and became the "nursing record". Once the fever treatment was finished, the handwritten nurses' notes in the fever charts were subsequently typewritten and forwarded to the psychiatrists whose secretaries then re-typed the notes, adding the name of the psychiatrists responsible for the treatment and filing them into the medical record. A carbon copy was filed in the record of the Fever Unit. The typewritten notes in the medical record became the official reports of the fever treatment. It is only due to the fact that the Ontario Hospital, Toronto retained the original records from its Fever Unit are we able to analyze the notes taken by the nurses. All the other nurses' notes have been destroyed and only so-called special reports (particularly related to restraints and forced treatments) have sometimes be conserved in the records. An analysis of the medical record and, in particular, the nurses' notes enables our understanding of how the fever treatment was used in psychiatric practice and how the "nurse technicians" applied this form of treatment. We illustrate our argument through the analysis of one record that we randomly picked from the list of treatments conducted in 1943.

Table 1: Treatment by gender, year, number and hours of treatment

Year		male	female	gender not speci-fied in record	total
1943	Patients	71	37	6	114
	Treatments	835	436	42	1313
	Hours	4073	2216 ¾	200 ¾	6490 ½
1944	Patients	46	19	2	67
	Treatments	432	174	22	628
	Hours	1970	833	105	2908
1945	Patients	45	27	1	73
	Treatments	461	229	1	691
	Hours	2001 ¼	1069 ¾	0	3071
1946	Patients	49	15	1	65
	Treatments	457	145	1	603
	Hours	2179	680	5	2864
1947	Patients	42	14	5	51
	Treatments	420	117	30	567
	Hours	2006 ¾	567 ½	131	2705 ¼
1948	Patients	37	13	2	52
	Treatments	301	134	22	457
	Hours	1367	639 ¼	84 ¼	2090 ½

An Overview of neuro-syphilis – its diagnostic, treatment, and the Kettering Hyphertherms

Neuro-syphilis (also termed general paresis) in all its different forms was a major public health concern in the first half of the twentieth century. According to Ontario psychiatrist C. M. Crawford, in 1921 approximately 20 percent of the admissions to Ontario psychiatric asylums were patients diagnosed with paresis.[3] Economists began to calculate the economic loss for the nation after the end of World War I as a result of neuro-syphilis. In 1918, the American statistician H. M. Pollock calculated that the "maintenance of the 1,554 patients with syphilitic insanity [in the state of New York – T. F] for a year would amount to $471,918.72"[4] and the loss of earnings of males would be $4,652,942.93 and that of females $273,782.92. Therefore, following Pollock,

3   Crawford (1921).
4   Pollock (1918), p. 278.

the total loss would account for $5,398,644.99.[5] Eleven years later, Pollock calculated that the "estimated economic loss on account of general paresis cases [one of the diagnostic terms for neuro-syphilis] are $15,757,008, and for cerebral syphilis cases [another diagnostic term for neuro-syphilis – T. F.] $813,588, making the total loss for the syphilitic group $16,570,596".[6] According to these calculations, the total loss had nearly tripled within 11 years. For psychiatrists, neuro-syphilis became one of the profession's major preoccupations not only because of the economic impact of the disease on national wealth, but also since it was the only psychiatric disorder for which psychiatrists were able to point out a biological cause. They claimed the ability to treat this disease in the same way somatic medicine was able to treat other diseases.

Serological tests

Much earlier in 1857, two German clinicians, F. von Esmarch and P. W. Jessen, determined that syphilis was the cause of general paresis and in 1905, F. R. Schaudin and E. Hoffmann described the spirocheta pallida as the pathogen of syphilis. In 1906, A. Wassermann, A. Neisser and C. Bruck introduced the so-called Wassermann test that became the standard test for neuro-syphilis.[7] Psychiatrists praised the Wassermann test for its reliability and by 1920, it was applied to nearly every new admission to a psychiatric asylum, becoming a kind of mass-screening instrument. For example, between 1937 and 1940, over 31 percent of the city of Chicago's entire adult population underwent Wassermann tests.[8] The test was performed with cerebral spinal fluid (CSF), which required a lumbar puncture, and in the case of a positive test, it was assumed that the CSF contained the spirocheta[9]. However, since its "discovery", many serologists raised serious objections against the test; the main objection being that it was too unspecific and positive reactions were obtained with patients suffering from multiple other clinical conditions (e. g. inflammations stemming from meningitis and diseases such as tuberculosis).[10]

Ludwik Fleck's important study (1935) about the construction of scientific facts through what he called thought collectives used the example of the Wassermann test to demonstrate how the test helped to make syphilis a scientific fact. In a chapter about the Wassermann reaction, Fleck emphasized the test's unreliability by noting that "one could achieve a positive Wassermann test with a normal blood sample and a negative result with a luetic [syphilitic –

5   Pollock (1918).
6   Pollock (1929), p. 195.
7   Crawford (1921).
8   Brandt (1988).
9   The mechanism of the Wassermann test can be simplified to an antigen-antibody reaction with cardiolipin as its antipbody. Larrañaga de/Trombetta/Wingeyer/Remondino (2006).
10 See, for example, Malcolm (1927); Schaffle/Riesenberg (1929); Scott/Reynolds (1944).

T. F.] blood sample without having committed any major technical mistake".[11] It was for this reason that serologists tried to develop other screening tests, including the Kahn test and the colloid gold test. Nonetheless, in Ontario the Wassermann test (sometimes combined with the Kahn test) was the standard one used in all psychiatric asylums at that time. All of these tests followed the Wassermann mechanism and, therefore, little to no variation in the degree of accurate diagnoses occurred. This fact is important to bear in mind for our later discussion of the fever treatment, as it puts into perspective both the psychiatrists' claims about the magnitude of neuro-syphilis as a public health issue and their claims about the success of their treatments, often "proven" by negative Wassermann tests.[12] At the Ontario Hospital, Toronto, many patients were treated in the fever unit even though their Wassermann test results were negative. Moreover, many of the patients treated as a result of a positive Wassermann test still tested positive once their treatment ended; the Wassermann test was interpreted rather arbitrarily.

Chemical treatments

With the "discovery" of the spirocheta pallida came the intensified search for treatment of neuro-syphilis. The first treatments were injections of mercury preparations. In 1910, "after 605 successive failures"[13] the German bacteriologist P. Ehrlich discovered "compound 606" to which he referred as Salvarsan – "the magic bullet"[14]. It was an arsephenamine, an arsenic compound that caused much pain upon injection, as did the mercury preparations. Whereas mercurial injections let to serious heavy metal toxicity in patients and left them "sweating and salivating, their tongues lacerated, teeth loosened by softened gum tissue, stomachs and bowels irritated, and bones so weakened that their noses collapsed jaws crumbled", arsenic injections caused irritations, abscesses and gangrene.[15] Tryparsamide, another arsenic compound used in psychiatry, was known as leading to "optic nerve disturbances which may result in blindness".[16] Despite these serious "side-effects", the combined use of arsenic, alongside mercury and bismuth, became from the 1920s the norm for the treatment of neuro-syphilis.[17] Actually, these arsenic compounds (there were a multitude of different arsenic compounds used in asylums in

---

11   Fleck (1980), p. 72.
12   See, for example, the review of the diagnostic accuracy of the Wassermann test at the Boston City Hospital by Patterson/Vilensky/Robertson/Berger (2012).
13   Young (2015), p. Loc 3398.
14   Verhave (2011), p. 3.
15   Young de (2015), p. Loc 3398.
16   Bromley: Artificial Fever Therapy (1939), n. p.
17   Thompson (1920). Detractors accused "Ehrlich of criminal negligence for aggressively marketing the drug for personal profit and for forcing prostitutes to undergo treatment at Frankfurt hospital" (Young de [2015], p. Loc 3398). However, Ehrlich developed neo-salvarsan that became the treatment of choice well into the mid-twentieth century.

Ontario), as well as all the other chemicals, were not able to cross the blood-brain barrier and, therefore, could not influence neuro-syphilis. Nevertheless, psychiatrists used them extensively and provided "evidence" for their effectiveness by referring to the different serological tests. The "chemical therapy" had to be administered over a period of 18 months.[18] These injections were extensively used in psychiatry. For example, at the Manitoba Government Clinic at St Boniface in Winnipeg in 1937, the arsenic compound called Mapharsen, the same one used in the Ontario Hospital, Toronto; 1,814 injections were given to 99 patients during four months in 1936.[19] These numbers are comparable to the number of injections given in Ontario asylums (these numbers were reported in the annual reports at the beginning of the 1930s).[20]

Psychiatrists were well aware of the life-threatening consequences of the chemicals used in the war against neuro-syphilis. Medical textbooks openly discussed the negative effects of the treatments, including the one published by the Ontario physician L. W. Harrison (1925).

Fever treatments and malaria fever therapy

Since the late-nineteenth century, psychiatrists experimented to treat paretic neuro-syphilis by the induction of fever. It was well known that the behaviours of patients diagnosed with psychoses changed when they came down with bacterial infections accompanied by high fever. Psychiatrists speculated that neuro-syphilis, caused by a bacterium, could similarly and successfully be treated by fever (and they imagined that it would be possible to treat other types of "insanity" which were not caused by bacteria). Psychiatrists used "the intravenous or intramuscular injection of various substances [to] provoke a general constitutional reaction which was frequently followed by clinical betterment".[21] The authors emphasized "clinical betterment" which means that

---

18 Kruif (1943).
19 Peterson (1937).
20 For example, at the Ontario Hospital, Brockville 2,354 injections had been administered in 1932 (with 137 first admissions due to general paresis) (Hospital Division Department of Mental Health [1934]), ranging from compounds like Mercurosal (a mercurial preparation) (Cole/Driver/Hutton [1922]), Tryparsemide (an arsenic preparation) (W. H. Brown / Pearce [1924]; Ebaugh/Dickson [1924]) and Novarsan (again an arsenic preparation). At Hamilton, the Annual Report mentions Ephedrine Hydrochloride in Catatonic stages, Cholesterol in Schizophrenia, Insulin in undernourished conditions, Carbon Dioxide in Schizophrenia. The Kingston asylum administered malaria inoculations, sulpholeum and tryparsamide injections. 560 manganese chloride injections had been given to "schizophrenic" (this is how psychiatrists called patients diagnosed with schizophrenia) but the psychiatrist noted "no clear cut mental changes". At the Ontario Hospital, Toronto (Queen Street) blood examinations in all suspected cases were performed, 30 malaria treatments, 800 iv. [intravenous – T. F.] injections of salvarsan or norvasan were administered, and 100 patients were treated with manganese chloride – 1700 injections in all (Hospital Division Department of Mental Health [1932]).
21 Bromberg (1936), p. 1184.

the patients' behaviour changed – a notion that was often used by psychiatrists to justify their "treatments". Among the substances with which psychiatrists experimented and which they used up into the late 1930s were intravenous typhoid vaccine, rat-bite fever, relapsing fever, intramuscular injections of sulphur, or of boiled milk, etc. Many of the substances were also used in the 1930s in Ontario psychiatric asylums: typhoid inoculations, diphteria toxoid, milk[22], or "Sulphur in Olive Oil"[23]. One of the physicians who experimented extensively with a wide array of substances was the Austrian physician Julius Wagner-Jauregg. Wagner-Jauregg received the Nobel Prize for Physiology or Medicine in 1927 for the fever therapy of neuro-syphilis, despite charges had been laid against him. He was dismissed after World War I for the maltreatment of soldiers.[24] He began injecting patients at the Clinic for Psychiatry and Nervous diseases with the streptococcus bacterium that causes erysipelas, or St. Anthony's Fire, that produced skin lesions and fever. Wagner-Jauregg later reflected upon his early trials with erysipelas as "an unfortunate experiment" that he "hardly had the authority then to carry on with".[25] The next step in his experimentations was the induction of tuberculin fever by injecting a recently developed vaccine to neuro-syphilitic asylum patients. It was only after alarming reports emerged about its toxic and fatal effects that he abandoned these experiments and began to use malaria-induced fevers. In 1917, Wagner-Jauregg took blood from a soldier with tertian malaria, a rarely fatal type of malaria, and injected it into a patient with neuro-syphilis.

> After an incubation period of about a week, the patients experienced chills and nausea, followed by raging fevers of more than 106° that lasted several hours. Over the next several days, fever alternated with chills until the patients were administered quinine sulfate to terminate the malarial infection. After a period of high fevers he administered quinine to end the malaria[26].

Although the malaria fever therapy "killed a number of these poor wretches who anyway were doomed"[27], it spread quickly across the world and became the standard treatment for neuro-syphilis in many countries. Asylums cultivated their own stock of malaria germs (*Plasmosium vivax*) by extracting blood from infected patients and using it to infect another group of neurosyphilitic patients. Psychiatrists also continued to induce fever in patients with other types of insanity, particularly schizophrenia, using an array of febrile agents. However, from the psychiatrists' perspective, the malaria fever therapy also had disadvantages and several complicating factors:

22 See, for example, Hospital Division Department of Mental Health (1934).
23 Bromley: Artificial Fever Therapy (1939), n.p. Another method that became "popular in the treatment of paresis consisted of threading some horsehair through the chest wall of the pitiable patient: an infection invariably resulted, followed by a large and painful abscess, and (although the mechanism was not understood at the time) the patient generally improved as a result of high fever which he developed" (Bromberg [1936], p. 1184).
24 Young (2015), p. Loc. 3689.
25 Eghigian (2010), p. 262.
26 Young de (2015), p. Loc 3672.
27 Kruif (1942), p. 11.

(1) The tertian parasite failed to give high fevers after repeated blood inoculations; (2) ethical considerations against injecting blood from one paretic to the other forced the institutions to start rearing and infecting mosquitoes for the transmission of the malaria parasite to patients, a rather specialistic (sic) job; (3) blacks responded poorly to *P. vivax* and for them the much more risky *P. falciparum* had to be used; and (4) salvarsan could not be used along with malaria infection because it also killed these parasites, but only as a follow-up treatment.[28]

Artificial fever and the Kettering Hypertherm

Due to these complicating factors and the urgent demands of the US Public Health Services for a quicker, "more effective method of wiping out the contagion by completing treatment rapidly in a hospital"[29], psychiatrists and engineers experimented with other methods to induce artificial fever in patients diagnosed with neuro-syphilis. The studies were carried out in close co-operation with industry, medicine and with frequent participation of the military. A research project led to the development of an apparatus in which the patient was put between two large plates and when the current was turned on the radio short-waves raised the patient's body temperature. After the development of the "radiotherm", Charles Franklin Ketterling, Vice President of General Motors, in conjunction with the Fever Research Project at the Miami Valley Hospital in Dayton, Ohio, began a series of experiments to improve the radiotherm. The "radio apparatus" had many serious defects. For example, whenever a pool of perspiration collected on any part of the patient's body, so called "eddy currents" would arc through this area and cause a severe skin burn.[30] P. de Kruif regularly took part in the experiments. "I was the first guinea pig, having the hell burned out of myself in the first crude air-conditioned GM radiotherm".[31] In the 1930s, the research group around Kettering invented what they called "the hypertherm".

In 1937, with the assistance of its Frigidaire Division, General Motors manufactured and furnished on loan 100 machines to asylums in North America and Europe.[32] Some psychiatrists enthusiastically celebrated the artificially-induced fever treatment as a breakthrough in the treatment of neuro-syphilis, one of them being Dr. A. J. Bromley of the Ontario Hospital, Toronto. Others were much more reluctant including "eminent specialists as Dr. Joseph Moore, of Baltimore, Maryland, and Dr. Paul O'Leary of Rochester, Minnesota" who opposed the assumption that "the results with artificial or physically induced fever therapy are as good, if not better, than those attained with malaria plasmodia or other infectious agents".[33]

---

28 Verhave (2011), p. 3, original italics.
29 Kruif (1943), p. 105.
30 Bromberg (1936), pp. 1185–1186; Simpson (1935).
31 Kruif, as cited in Verhave (2011), p. 3.
32 Kruif (1937).
33 Bromberg (1936), p. 1187.

In the remainder of this chapter, we critically question the narrative that "the fever machine had saved thousands of lives and had prevented the spread of syphilis from which infected people would have otherwise languished in a miserable state of body and mind".[34]

Fever Treatment in Action

Based on the Fever Unit documents examined, we can assume that the decision to invest in the "temperature cabinets" (the official term used at the Ontario Hospital, Toronto) was made after due consideration and consultations with the Ontario Minister of Health Harold James Kirby (1937–1942). Dr. A.J. Bromley, who was appointed to staff in 1938 as graduate medical intern[35], and Dr. H. W. Hills from the Department of the Provincial Secretary visited in mid-August 1939 six mental hospitals, three general hospitals, one US state prison and the Department of Physiotherapy at Northwestern University (all institutions in the states of Michigan and Illinois) on behalf of the Ministry of Health to evaluate the potential benefits of this form of treatment. On 29 August 1939, Bromley wrote a letter and a detailed report of this travel to the Minister of Health. Before describing his conclusions in more detail, Bromley emphasized that he had "been guided by a study of a large number of reports which have appeared in medical literature during the past few years".[36] The last statement is important to bear in mind for the analysis of the patient records given that all of the preventive measures recommended in the literature had not been implemented in the Ontario asylum.

Bromley was one of the chief advocates of this Fever Unit. From the patient records and all of the records related to the Fever Unit, it is obvious that Bromley played a central role in the fever treatment application. In his letter, he argued that even though physical fever

> has not yet been used for a sufficient length of time for statistical records to be of very great value, it would appear that the results obtained with it in the treatment of neurosyphilis are at least comparable to those resulting from malarial inoculations and may be 20% or 25% better.[37]

Bromley claimed that this form of treatment was "perfectly controllable at all time". The mode of action of the fever treatment was unknown, nonetheless he concluded that physical fever "would seem to have a definite place in the treatment of neurosyphilis[...] [and] offers to the patient [...] increased safety and comfort".[38]

According to Bromley, physical fever would make it possible to treat patients even without admitting them and without their being forced to disrupt

---

34 Verhave (2011), p. 4.
35 Hospital Division Department of Mental Health (1938).
36 Bromley: Artificial Fever Therapy (1939), n. p.
37 Bromley: Artificial Fever Therapy (1939), n. p.
38 Bromley: Artificial Fever Therapy (1939), n. p.

their working life. Furthermore, the course of the treatment was totally under the control of the psychiatrists, whereas one characteristic of malaria treatment was that the infection could only be stopped by quinine. Bromley therefore concluded that physical fever should be considered the treatment of choice.

In his letter to the Minister, Bromley does not withhold the fact that he considered fever therapies as "with a certain danger to the patients". The death rate for malaria therapy ranges, according to the author, "from 3 % in very carefully selected patient, up as high as 30 %, according to some authors. Physical fever is said to show a death rate of about 2 %." Nevertheless, Bromley stated that chemical therapy and artificial fever should be combined.[39]

As previously mentioned, the letter to the Minister was accompanied by a detailed report about the administration of the artificial fever treatment in different institutions. We focus on one section of the report that concerns the description of the visit to the South Michigan State Prison. The description highlights some aspects that prove illuminating in our later discussion of the disciplinary dimension of the artificial fever treatment.

Bromley began his report about the State Prison by describing the population of

> about 5,000 prisoners, practically all of whom have been sentenced to long terms of imprisonment. Over 10 % (525) of their population is suffering from syphilis. Of these 525 cases 17 ½ [sic] have positive spinal fluids. All inmates have blood Wassermann reactions following admission and where these reactions are positive, cerebral spinal fluid reactions are obtained; in addition, *any inmate whose neurological examination, or whose behaviour inside of the prison suggests the advisability. Only a very small percentage of the prisoners are definitely psychotic. Most of those treated by artificial fever are cases of asymptomatic neurosyphilis.*[40]

This quote is revealing in that it underscores that many prisoners were treated as a result of "their behaviour inside the prison" and not due to their presumed serological values or their being "definitely psychotic". It does suggest that most of the prisoners were "treated" for disciplinary considerations. Furthermore, Bromley emphasized that artificial fever was "used here very extensively" with three cabinets in operation (using the much more dangerous) "high frequency electromagnetic induction."

> During the past 21 months, about 4,000 treatments have been given, totalling over 21,000 hours of fever above 105 degrees. The treatments are administered by inmates whose recordings of temperature, pulse, cabinet temperature, etc., are checked from time to time by one of the guards. A doctor is usually in the prison when treatments are being given but may be at a considerable distance from the fever therapy department and not immediately available. At time, it is said, a doctor may not visit the treatment unit at all during the day, but ordinarily one of the medical staff looks in from time to time.[41]

By describing the treatments in this way, Bromley gave the impression that the administration of the fever treatments was without any danger and that every-

---

39   Bromley: Artificial Fever Therapy (1939).
40   Bromley: Report (1939), n. p., emphasis added.
41   Bromley: Report (1939), emphasis added.

one could administer it – even prisoners or guards with a short period of training. All in all, according to Bromley, the artificial fever treatment was "a very safe procedure, only 3 deaths having occurred which might be ascribed to the effects of the fever" and even "men over 60 years have been treated". Again, the description provided by Bromley contradicts not only the life-threatening incidences that regularly occurred in the administration of the fever treatments at the Ontario Hospital, Toronto, but also all the medical literature of the time. However, we want to point out once again that Bromley was well aware of the disciplining dimension of this form of treatment. He emphasized that

> [a]s in most other places were artificial fever is in use, they report clinical improvement in psychotic cases and improved behavior in unco-operative patients occurring very quickly after treatment started. Serology does not usually change for a considerable length of time and many patients receive over 100 hours of treatment, some as much as 175 hours.[42]

Bromley reported about a man who "had been constantly in trouble with the authorities for infraction of the prison regulations; he admitted this and said that since he had been on fever therapy he had had no trouble and his head felt much clearer".[43]

Bromley appears to have been successful in his campaign. Although we have not been able to retrieve the complete administrative records about the purchase of these cabinets, we have been able to trace the investment. A memorandum from 1940 outlines the equipment needed to furnish the unit and the corresponding prices for these items.[44] From our research, we note that in January 1940 psychiatrists began to "screen" the patient population of the Ontario Hospital, Toronto in order to treat in the Fever Unit only those patients who would appear to have had the greatest chance of success. For every admitted patient with the diagnosis of neuro-syphilis, the biography in the record was summarized on half a page and these typewritten summaries (all dated January 16, 1940) were classified as "unsuitable" cases[45] and "suitable" cases. The classification "unsuitable" was apparently only attributed to patients who had already been treated unsuccessfully with multiple other chemicals and/or fever treatments. These patients also stood out due to their "aggressive" or "violent" behaviour, or who had been in the asylum for many years.[46]

---

42 Bromley: Report (1939).
43 Bromley: Report (1939), n. p.
44 No author (1940). This document suggests that Bromley proposed not to buy the fever cabinet but rather to purchase pre-fabricated parts to assemble the cabinet at the hospital. This approach would reduce the financial investment needed (and we speculate, make the decision to invest more acceptable). The Annual Report of 1940 states that the fever cabinet was successfully assembled in the hospital.
45 Unsuitable cases (1940).
46 We retrieved the patient records of 11 randomly chosen patients from the list of "unsuitable cases" to develop an understanding of the rationale behind the decision to consider

The way in which patients were screened for the fever treatment contradicts Bromley's claim that this form of treatment was successful in patients who had been treated without success with other fever treatments. We would argue that psychiatrists at the early stages of the Fever Unit's operation only chose those cases which would "prove" the success of the new form of treatment. The screening was obviously not used to exclude patients with somatic conditions who could be endangered by the fever treatment. For example, Carl H., who had been admitted in 1933, was suffering from "a heart condition" but had to undergo the treatment despite this diagnosis.[47] This finding contradicts another of Bromley's claims, namely that patients should be assessed carefully as to their physical condition, and, in particular their heart condition in order to exclude patients who may have suffered from a heart condition. On 21 February 1941, roughly one year after the list of "unsuitable cases" had been written, psychiatrists prepared another list entitled "List of Neurosyphilitis Patients who are discharged or on probation following treatment and are adjusting satisfactorily (1941)".[48] One of our case examples, Carmen B., appeared on this list. The list includes 48 "successful" cases treated in the Fever Unit in one year. However, in examining the corresponding medical records, it is apparent that the psychiatrists' judgements did not always meet the perceptions of the patients' family members and very often, the "successful cases" had been re-admitted later.

One example is William W. who had been admitted to the Ontario Hospital, Toronto on 7 March 1940 with the diagnosis neuro-syphilis, treated with the artificial fever treatment, and discharged on 24 December 1940 after probation. The medical record includes a considerable number of letters that are obviously responses to letters from William's spouse. However, from the response letters, it is clear that his spouse wrote her letters to account or report to the psychiatrists, a normal procedure at that time when patients were on probation. These reports often described in detail the patient's behaviour at home and enabled the psychiatrist to maintain control over the patient even after discharge. From the psychiatrists' response letters, it becomes clear that William's spouse did not believe that the treatment had been successful and asked for her husband to be re-admitted a couple of months after the probation period ended, which the psychiatrists refused.[49] Nevertheless, despite the

---

these cases as "unsuitable". The Casebook numbers for these patients are 59129, 18886, 19568, 22482, 19379, 195852, 25882, 21597, 12504, 20649 and 28433.

47   Carl H. patient record 20649.

48   The list contains 48 names and we pulled every third name to retrieve their medical records and to analyze the case history in the records. In the event that we could not retrieve one of the records we went to the next one (fourth instead of third and so on). All in all we pulled 16 medical records (Casebook numbers: 22699, 22905, 23145, 23429, 23671, 22834, 23271, 23183, 23313, 22937, 23002, 22534, 22587, 22686, 22415, 22548, 56654) (List of Neurosyphilitis Patients who are discharged or on probation following treatment and are adjusting satisfactorily [1941]).

49   William W. patient record 23002.

continuous complaints of his spouse, William was referenced in the list from 1941 as a successful case.

A similar case was that of Peter M. who is listed as being successfully treated but the letters from his spouse tell a different story.[50] We provide these two examples to emphasize that what psychiatrists classified as "successful" treatments was at a minimum questionable. In our opinion, this list was compiled with the aim to justify further investments in the unit and to demonstrate the success of this form of treatment. Our findings, therefore, suggest that psychiatrists systematically exaggerated the "success story" of fever treatments, which would also challenge the numbers of successful treatments published in the literature.

Regardless, the Fever Unit at the Ontario Hospital, Toronto became the referral centre to which other Ontario asylums transferred their patients.[51] In 1943, the unit had more than four temperature cabinets.[52] In what follows, we present how nurses applied the fever treatments and demonstrate that artificial fever treatments systematically put patients' lives in danger. We begin by describing the significance of the Fever Unit in the treatment of neuro-syphilis in Ontario. Using two individual cases, we then describe the "fever treatments in action".

As mentioned at the beginning of the article a sharp decline in patients treated in the Fever Unit occured in 1944, which might be partly due to the introduction of penicillin in 1943. Penicillin had contributed to the decline of syphilis in the USA from a high of 72 cases per 100,000 in 1943 to about 4 per 100,000 in 1956.[53] Nevertheless, it is noteworthy that the Unit persisted into the 1950s, long after penicillin had been introduced in the treatment of syphilis. At the Ontario Hospital, Toronto, fever therapy had even been combined with penicillin (AR, 1949).[54]

Fever treatment in action

The physiological effects of fever

In a manual written by Bromley in 1940 and obviously aimed at instructing nurses (or nurse-technicians as they were called in the literature[55]), the course

---

50   Peter M. patient record [two records with different casebook numbers: 23249 and 23671].
51   Hospital Division Department of Mental Health (1941).
52   Fever Unit Treatments (monthly) (1943–1954).
53   Brown, W.J. (1970).
54   Hospitals Division Department of Health (1950).
55   By 1909, psychiatric nursing had been recognized as a nursing specialization in the province of Ontario. Nurses employed by the Ontario Hospital, Toronto, at the time of this study, underwent a 12-week training program administered by a psychiatrist (see, also, Tipliski (2004)). We have no specific information of the nurses' training in the fever unit. From the literature, we know that in 1936 the procedure was considered so dangerous to the patients that the manufacturer for this reason decided to only use the "fever

of a fever therapy treatment was set at a total of 50 hours of fever over 105 degrees Fahrenheit, given in treatments of six or seven hours' duration, once or twice weekly. In this paper, Bromley also recognized that the mode of action of the "treatment" could not be explained. It was well known that it was not possible, according to Bromley, to kill off the spirochaete (considered the cause of syphilis) in the human body by artificial fever because the thermo-lethal point for the parasite is about 112 degrees F and the human body cannot be heated to such a degree. The "low fever" therefore was not able to kill the germs, so arsenic compounds (Tryparsemide, Mapharsan, and Bismuth) were given simultaneously.[56]

In a section titled "Physiological Effects of Fever", Bromley provided a list with 16 "important physiological phenomena that are found associated with artificial fever". This list puts into perspective Bromley's former claims of fever treatments as "perfectly controllable at all time" – the "physiological effects" must be considered as serious, life-threatening events. Not only would the heart rate increase (to about 130 to 140 beats per minute) but "actually a temporary cardiac decompensation occurs at these temperatures, due to the inadequate filling of the heart because of the shortened filling time". The increased and deepened respiration "may occasionally be severe enough to lead to an alkalosis"[57] and "frequently some cyanosis[58] [is] present". The "basal metabolic rate [...] increases of about 50% over the normal"[59] and the "blood pressure falls" sometimes resulting in "vasomotor collapse"[60]. Furthermore, the treatment leads to "a marked stimulation of leukocytosis[61] [...] and an increase of all the cellular constituents of the blood if concentration from dehydration occurs"[62]. Additionally, a great "increase in perspiration, with a result-

---

machines" at their research unit. In an article in the Journal of Nursing (1936), Bromberg wrote that "[t]he production and maintenance of artificial fever therapy at high temperature is not adaptable to ordinary office practice. The physicians and nurses charged with this undertaking receive special training in the Department of Fever Therapy Research at the Miami Valley Hospital before the apparatus is released. Adequate preliminary training of physician personnel and nurse personnel is an essential requirement for this type of work" (Bromberg (1936), p. 1186). Nursing journals also reported about the fever treatment, see, for example, Lehmann (1937); Lutz (1936).

56   Bromley (1940).
57   "If not immediately treated, alkalosis on its own can develop into a life-threatening condition." Hadjiliadis (2014); Martin (2015).
58   "Cyanosis can be a sign of a beginning shock. Shock is a life-threatening condition that occurs when the body is not getting enough blood flow. As many as 1 in 5 people who suffer shock will die from it." Borke (2015); Hadjiliadis (2015).
59   "The basal metabolic rate, or BMR, is a measure of the rate at which a person's body "burns" energy, in the form of calories, while at rest." Dowshen (2015).
60   Vasomotor collapse is used as another term for shock (see footnote 55).
61   Leukocytosis refers to an increase in the total number of white blood cells (WBCs).
62   The increase of WBCs and the simultaneous decrease of the liquid component of the blood (due to the excessive sweating) makes the blood "thicker" aggravating the scenario described in footnote 55. Another life-threatening condition as a result of the changed blood composition is the development of edema, which is an excess of watery fluid collecting in the cavities or tissues of the body.

ing loss of sodium chloride"[63] occurs, leading to the loss of "4000 cc's or more of sweat"; "[i]t has been shown that there is a constant anoxia[64] during fever, and [...] [e]vidence of tetany[65] occasionally occurs in patients"; the absorption "of fluid from the intestinal tract is inhibited during high fever"; and "[o]cca-sionally, mild delirium may occur".[66] This list puts into perspective Bromley's claim that this form of treatment was a harmless intervention that could be performed by anyone with basic training, as in the case of the US State Prison that Bromley used as an example. Bromley's list highlights that these treat-ments affected all organs and bodily functions and as our empirical research demonstrates, this list is a significant understatement of what actually hap-pened with patients during artificial fever treatments.

In another section of the paper, Bromley provided an overview of "Com-plications met with in the Fever Therapy". He emphasized the need for "alert attention by a well-trained nurse-technician" because "two great dangers in fever" needed to "be kept constantly in mind. The first is disturbance of the heat-regulation mechanism of the body, resulting if unheeded, in heat-stroke[67]. The second is circulatory collapse"[68]. However, Bromley claimed that the oc-currence of these complications was so rare that it could practically be ne-glected, or at least easily be compensated for.

In 68 of the 451 case files from the Fever Unit, the treatment was inter-rupted due to life-threatening incidents. In short, in 15 percent of the cases, the patients nearly died and no clear indication of what happened after their referral to their respective ward exists. In some instances, these patients appar-ently suffered severe damage, as for example when nurses noted "cerebral accident" or "cerebral incident".[69] Our analysis demonstrates that in 52.7 per-cent of the cases treated at the Fever Unit the treatment never reached at even

---

63 Complications of severe and rapidly developing hyponatremia may include cerebral edema (swelling of the brain), seizures, coma, and brain damage. Acute or severe hypona-tremia may be fatal without prompt and appropriate medical treatment Higdon (2001).

64 "[A]noxia is a condition in which there is an absence of oxygen supply ... In severe cases of anoxia, ... the patient is often stuperous or comatose (in a state of unconsciousness) for periods ranging from hours to days, weeks, or months. Seizures, myoclonic jerks (muscle spasms or twitches), and neck stiffness may occur ... Mental changes such as dementia or a psychosis may occur. Mental confusion, personality regression, parietal lobe syn-dromes, amnesia, hallucinations, and memory loss may also occur" (National Institute of Neurological Disorders and Stroke [n. y.]).

65 "Tetany ... is characterized by spasms of the hands and feet, cramps, spasm of the voice box (larynx), and overactive neurological reflexes. Tetany is generally considered to re-sult from very low calcium levels in the blood" (MedicineNet [2016]).

66 All citations from Bromley (1940), pp. 2–3.

67 Heatstroke is where the body is no longer able to cool itself and a person's body tempera-ture becomes dangerously high. It can put a strain on the brain, heart, lungs, liver and kidneys, and can be life-threatening. Symptoms of heat stroke can include confusion, agitation, disorientation, the absence of sweating, and coma.

68 Bromley (1940), pp. 6–7.

69 See, for example, Bernado A. patient record number 25870; David G. patient record number 25451.

5 hours, being discontinued due to the occurrence of uncontrollable events. Furthermore, our analysis highlights that none of the patients treated in the Fever Unit received the "medically indicated" series of treatment. Neither regarding the length of the treatments nor the number of treatments (the course of a fever therapy was set at a total of 50 hours of fever over 105 degrees Fahrenheit, given in treatments of six or seven hours' duration). According to our findings the treatments were rather randomly applied.

The medical literature shows that all these effects were well known including warnings of increased death risk. Patients experienced weight loss during treatment (5 kilograms) but specific risks also existed during the induction phase.[70] Gore and Isaacson (1949) summarized the research undertaken between 1927 and 1947 reporting the dangers, particularly changes in blood serology that had been well studied. These authors also underscored that most deaths occurred days after the interruption of the treatment and that "it is nearly impossible to control and predict the risks of collapse" which leads to most deaths, emphasizing an "increased risk of complications after the treatment".[71] Considering that Bromley emphasized in his initial letter to the Ontario Minister of Health that he had "been guided by a study of a large number of reports which have appeared in medical literature during the past few years"[72], it is surprising that he never mentioned the results of these studies. Bromley was well aware of the research undertaken up to 1939, yet he was obviously not concerned about the serious "side effects" of the treatment and systematically downplayed the risks for the patients. Even some of Bromley's colleagues warned at the beginnings of the 1930s of sudden temperature increases in some patients and that "apparently no method of recognizing such cases in advance" existed.[73] Others described patients who, "during the course of treatment, suddenly, and without warning, developed an extremely high temperature which could not be controlled, and died".[74] In some cases, "fever therapy had to be discontinued because of the development of such untoward symptoms as shock, coma, convulsions, or hyperexcitability [...] [and] deaths occurred in cases in which *symptoms developed from 2 to 36 hours following a fever treatment lasting from 3 to 11 hours*".[75] These symptoms are exactly those described in the nurses' notes. Moreover these findings are disturbing in that they indicate that more patients were killed by these treatments than has been assumed to date, especially as the "pathologic changes have never been clearly defined, although clinicians have long time be aware of the danger of high body temperature".[76]

---

70   H. R. Brown/Clark/Jones/Walther/Warren (1943).
71   H. R. Brown et al. (1943), pp. 474–475.
72   Bromley: Artificial Fever Therapy (1939), n. p.
73   McKay/Gray/Winans (1933); McKay/Winans (1932).
74   Telfer (1934), p. 16.
75   Gore/Isaacson (1949), p. 1032, emphasis added.
76   Gore/Isaacson (1949), p. 1039.

Furthermore, authors described a "maniacal state due to the pending collapse" in case of dehydration and "grand mal seizures, twitching, athetoid movements of arms and legs, etc." in case of overhydration. These patients "develop edema and become restless and emotional unstable".[77] Furthermore, the lack of oxygen (anoxia) leads to severe cellular defects[78] and to serious damages of all organs, to the central nervous system (CNS) and to complex anatomic changes in the brain,[79], which means that the fever treatments led to neuronal degeneration[80]. These comments highlight that the behaviour described by the nurses in their notes and used as evidence for the severity of the mental disease was actually (co-)produced by the treatment. Not only did this behaviour occur during the actual treatment, but the research emphasized that recovery was slow and the patients are in a "water logged state". Mental confusion and "irritability [persist – T. F.] for 2–7 days after treatment".[81] The authors agreed that giving caffeine and oxygen[82] during collapse was not effective, an aspect also underscored in the study by Gore and Isaacson (1949). Therefore, the emergency measures taken at the Ontario Hospital, Toronto were ineffective and patients who did survive the treatment needed days to readjust.

No preventive measure was ever initiated at the Fever Unit in the Ontario Hospital, Toronto, but rather Bromley denied any risks associated with this form of treatment. Our research into the Fever Unit demonstrates that these "complications" were an integral part of the treatment. Moreover, these life-threatening treatments were carried out despite the fact that psychiatrists at the time did not believe that they led to a cure, referring to patients treated solely as being in "remission".

Seen against the backdrop of what was known at that time about the physiological implications of artificial fever, the manner in which these treatments were carried out at the Ontario Hospital, Toronto appears to have been grossly negligent. Their administration violated existing recommendations as to how to use artificial fever treatments, but also was applied to groups of patients who should have been excluded according to existing consensus in the medical community, given their high risk of undergoing severe damage from these treatments. For example, one researcher warned to not administer artificial fever treatments to patients "past forty years of age".[83] However, at the Ontario Hospital, Toronto, patients over 60 years of age were still treated – with devastating effects, as in the case of Enrico C. who was treated in 1946 at the age of 68 years and the last nurse's note stated "despite supportive treatment – cerebral involvement feared".[84] The following section outlines how

77   Belt/Folkenberg (1940); Bromley (1940); Brown, H. R. et al. (1943).
78   See, for example, Barcroft (1920); Courville (1936); Gore/Isaacson (1949).
79   See, also, Hicks/Holt/Guerrant/Leavell (1948); Landis (1928).
80   Landis (1928).
81   Brown, H. R. et al. (1943), pp. 476–481.
82   See also Gore/Isaacson (1949); Hartman (1937).
83   Belt/Folkenberg (1940), p. 170.
84   Enrico C. patient record number 25760.

nurses applied the artificial fever and how they recorded the patients' behaviours and reactions to the treatment.

The Fever Unit at the Ontario Hospital, Toronto

In this section, we analyze in more detail a case selected randomly from the records preserved from the Fever Unit (described earlier). As noted, the nurses' notes were transcribed in medical notes thereby transforming them into a "sanitized" account of the events.

Stephen O.

Stephen O. (all names are pseudonyms), an immigrant from the former Yugoslavia, was transferred to the Ontario Hospital, Toronto on 15 September 1942 from the New Toronto asylum (the academic psychiatric asylum).[85] The anamnesis, taken nearly one month after Same O. had been admitted at New Toronto, stated that Stephen O. landed in 1925 in Quebec and "since that time worked on farms and for the last few years has worked in mines". He worked in a gold mine in Timmins from 1931 but started to act "quite queerly" in 1939, but no other information was available about his actions at work. According to his physician, who issued the certificate that led to Stephen O.'s compulsory admission, Stephen's "conversation was at times incoherent; he found difficulty in expressing himself and often repated (sic) what he said".

On 1 September 1942 the psychiatrist at New Toronto summarized the notes about Stephen O. in one paragraph titled "mental status." This definition then became Stephen O.'s official mental condition and, apart from the serological tests, the basis of his diagnosis.

> Behaviour and Appearance: This man is restless and untidy. At times he jumps out of bed and pulls the clothes off the mattress. He is overactive and confused. However, he is friendly and cooperative as he can be. His appetite is good. He sleeps well without sedative although he has been noisy on several occasions at night. He takes no particular interest in his environment and can not [sic] be persuaded to do any work about the ward. He shows little interest in the other patients although he complains about being near deteriorated patients and evidently realizes that they are mentally ill.

These comments are interesting insofar as the details provided must have been derived from the nurses' observations/notes that unfortunately are no longer part of the record. However, the observations about Stephen O.'s behaviour on the ward, e.g. "jumps out of bed and pulls clothes and mattress" or he is "overactive and confused", his appetite and his missing interest in his environment are observed and reported by the nurses. In particular, terms like "untidy" were terms that nurses used to describe patients who became

---

85   All information taken from: Stephen O. patient record 26599. We selected this record at random with no particular reason to choose it over the others in the files.

incontinent or refused to use the bathroom. Reading the psychiatrists' notes in this way enables one to conclude indirectly what the focus of the nurses was in writing down their observations. We demonstrate this connection in the cases where we have the nursing notes at our disposal.

Between Stephen O.'s admission at New Toronto and his transfer to the Ontario Hospital, Toronto many different serological tests were performed (Standard Khan test, Kolmer Wassermann test, Quantitative Khan test), all of which were positive and supported the diagnosis of neuro-syphilis. On 14 September 1942, Stephen O. was presented to the psychiatrists' regularly scheduled clinical conference. It was during these conferences that the diagnosis of a patient was determined and the course of treatment decided. However, in Stephen O.'s case, both diagnosis and treatment had been determined long before the conference. Already on 3 September, the superintendent from New Toronto wrote to the director of the "Fever Therapy Department" at the Ontario Hospital, Toronto requesting Stephen O.'s treatment at the Ontario Hospital, Toronto. The asylum agreed to admit Stephen O. to the Fever Unit and one day after the conference, Stephen O. was transferred to there. A copy of the medical record was send with the patient (the reason why we are able to access the notes prepared at New Toronto).

Practically no nursing notes have been conserved from Stephen O.'s admission and stay, apart from a document entitled "Ward Admission Record" and a "Report on Physical Condition". The nurses described Stephen O. in these forms as "talkative – co-operative" and "well nourished, clean, nor vermin". During the psychiatrists' clinical conference of 21 September 1942, it was reported that Stephen O. "was somewhat restless, talkative and elated. States he feels fine, that he never felt better. Conversation is rambling and disconnected." Concurring with a diagnosis of Psychosis with Syphilitic Meningo-Encephalitis, the psychiatrists sent him for fever therapy. On 24 September 1942, Stephen O. underwent a physical examination. What is remarkable about the physical examinations before fever treatments is their clear violation of the rigid guidelines for selecting patients and for administration of the treatment adopted by the American Medical Association (AMA) in 1934. The AMA recognized early "that fever therapy is not without danger, and rigid controls were adopted both in the selection of patients and in the method of administration".[86] Due to the massive pathologic changes in fever treatments, a thorough "physical examination, roentgenogram of the chest" (this step was done in the Ontario Hospital, Toronto), "blood count, chemical analysis of the blood, urinalysis and electrocardiogram" were requested.[87] All these precautionary measures were ignored in the Toronto asylum. After his treatments, Stephen O. was discharged in August 1943, but re-admitted five years later.

86   Gore/Isaacson (1949), p. 1030.
87   Gore/Isaacson (1949), pp. 1030–1031.

The life-threatening dimension of the fever treatments

We focus on the treatment from 17 November 1942 to demonstrate that life-threatening incidences during the fever treatment were no exception but rather an integral part of routine treatment. Up to this day, Stephen O. had received 33 ¾ hours of fever treatment at "over 105 °F". Often nurses noted what patients said "verbatim" (or at least what they thought was worth noting in the form of direct speech as it would prove the patient's madness) providing a glimpse of how the patient may have experienced certain situations. On 23 October 1942 the nurse in charge of Stephen O. noted "[s]peaks frequently" of "you're electrocuting me in this box, I die here. Still very difficult to reason with patient".[88] On 17 November 1942, the psychiatrist's note states

> 10th treatment. Took 3 hours. Patient was resistive and unco-operative throughout whole treatment. After 3 hours, temperature coasted suddenly. Patient cyanosed. Respiration ceased temporarily. Pulse became imperceptible. Oxygen was administered along with 1 amp. caffeine, sodium benzoate and 50 c.c. 50% glucose was terminated. 50 c.c. of 50% glucose was also administered every two hours throughout treatment. Condition on return to ward only fair. Patient is fairly well oriented and shows fair degree of insight. His judgement however, remains poor.

An analysis of the nurses' fever chart provides a more dramatic picture. The construction of the chart allows for very complex information to be comprehended at a glance.

The left side of the chart was reserved for reports on the patient's behaviour during the "treatment" and the intake of liquids. The scale in the middle of the chart shows the actual temperature of the machine (temperature cabinet). The left graph shows the pulse rate (bpm) of the patient during the treatment.

The right part of the chart contains a scale with the timeline of the treatment (on the far right), the medications given during the "treatment" and other "nursing interventions". The graph on the same side shows the patient's actual body temperature. The bottom of the chart includes on the left a summary of the observations of the patient's behaviour. On the right, the chart contains medical information about the patient's physical condition after the treatment.

In Stephen O.'s case, the nurses reported that during the "induction phase" the patient was "talkative asking for sedation". Knowing that the treatment was physiologically challenging in the induction phase, Bromley discussed a temporary heart decompensation at temperatures around 102 °F – the comment of Stephen O. being "talkative" indicates that the nurse had little comprehension of the patient's situation.[89] Similar remarks reinforce this point. Although the pulse appeared to be very unstable, the nurse noted at 9:45 that

---

88 Stephen O. patient record number 26599.

89 We should emphasize that we do not wish to speculate about the nurses' feelings in applying these treatments. Rather, we are arguing that the nurses treated these patients totally as a regular exercise. We do not wish to suggest that the nurses did not care, but

"restless hands out constantly" and at 10:00 "some part of body moving". Just at the moment that the patient experienced a cardiac crisis (the nurse noted at 11:15 pulse absent) she reported: "restless, resistive extremely noisy + resistive" and reacted by administering Pantopon (a sedative). Even when the pulse was absent, she did not discontinue the treatment, but waited 45 minutes until Stephen O. had a respiratory arrest (at 12:00). At 11:45, the nurse noted that she gave Caffeine Sodium Benzoate, glucose infusion, and later oxygen. Patient then "expectorates white mucus and vomits green fluid" – probably bile. The nurse's reaction countervailed Bromley's strict instruction that in cases of a "marked disproportion between temperature and pulse rate, or a tendency for the pulse rate to fall as the temperature rises [...] calls for cessation of treatment at once". However, her only comment at the end after this highly critical incident was that the patient was "resistive and uncooperative. No apparent change in mental condition". A similar incident occurred again only one week later on 24 November 1942 (Stephen O. received his treatments on a weekly basis). The treatment was again discontinued because Stephen O. had some type of cardiac event. This time the nurse noted that the volume of the pulse was weak. She administered glucose and sedated the patient with pantopon. However, she opened the cabinet due to the pulse losing volume.

> Very restless during entire treatment. Oriented in all spheres. Insight good. No hallucinations or delusions. B. P. prior to treatment was 100/64 and B. P. after treatment was 105/68. 3 1/5 hours temp over 105. Pulse – fair quality – losing volume after 3 hrs of treatment. color- flushed – slightly cyanosed after 3 hrs. Cond. on disch. [condition at discharge – T. F.] – satisfactory.[90]

Stephen O.'s record contains another intriguing document, a so-called treatment plan in which it is noted that he received "special treatment". No references exist to show what was meant by "special treatment" nor can we find any reports of them. However, from other records and minutes we do know that "special treatment" was a synonym for "shock treatment", probably Electro-Convulsive Therapy or ECT. This assumption is supported by the Annual Report of 1944:

> Electro-shock treatment has been found to be a useful preparatory treatment in cases of General Paresis, who are unco-operative because of excitement, or in poor physical condition from a depressive syndrome, and several cases have shown surprising mental improvement before starting the course of artificial fever treatment.[91]

This finding indicates that Stephen O. underwent treatment that could not be justified from a pathophysiological point of view. Rather, our research highlights that these fever treatments can only be understood if they are analyzed as part of a psychiatric "dispositive". Our assumption is also supported through the literature which frequently emphasized that the mechanisms of

---

rather that they were implicated in the scenario and did not share any empathy with the patients because they carried on with the treatments.

90   Stephen O. patient record number 26599.

91   Hospital Division Department of Health (1944).

the treatment could not be explained but that they had a "positive effect" on patients. It becomes particularly obvious in our next case example.

Connie B.

Connie B.'s case record is incomplete. A list of fever treatments carried out in the Ontario Hospital, Toronto indicates that her treatment was considered successful. The peculiarity of this record is that it contains many pages of nurses' notes about the "everyday" treatment on the ward. No fever chart actually exists from the Fever Unit, and few psychiatrists' documents survived. However, many daily or weekly nursing documents describing Connie B.'s treatments and her condition afterwards are available. Connie B., an Italian immigrant, was admitted on 26 October 1939. Her admission certificate stated that she was "wildly excited. Lying naked on floor. Screaming. A few days ago claimed to be divine and to bear the "bruises of Christ". No relevant answers but only talk of special revelations". After intensive continuous bath treatments combined with continuous packs (meaning that she was packed in wet bed sheets that became tight when drying up), tube feeding, restraints, and sedatives, she received her first "fever treatment" in December 1939. This treatment was discontinued, apparently because it was impossible to keep her in the machine. Connie B. spent nearly half of the time at the asylum in continuous bath, continuous packs, or restraint, and was tube fed most of this time. On 4 January 1940, Connie B. survived a cardiac arrest in the continuous pack. After this incident, she again endured a period of continuous baths/packs, as well as seclusion. Another course of fever treatment was carried out in October 1940 and she was discharged in May 1941. As was the case for the use of ECT, continuous baths were used independently of an individual diagnosis in all cases of disobedient and resistant patients, as all the records used for this analysis highlight. Again, continuous baths were not guided by a nosography or kind of medical-theoretical knowledge, but rather were techniques of discipline.

The disciplining character of continuous baths is recognized implicitly in the Annual Report of 1943: "Unfortunately we have been unable to operate the continuous bath because of the shortage of staff, and for the same reason it has been necessary to increase the amount of sedatives given to patients, especially at night".[92]

As already mentioned, Connie B. received her first fever treatment on 15 December 1939. According to the report the night before, she had voided, had been given enemas at 7:00 and 8:00 PM, had received Bromide as a sedative, and "orange juice with 2 tbsp glucose" – all as routine preparation for the fever treatment next day – but she remained "very uncooperative + resistive". Because she was "noisy-singing and talking" she was "placed in CWP [continuous water pack]". But even in the pack she was "noisy and disturbing the

92 Hospital Division Department of Health (1944), p. 15.

whole ward". She was kept in the pack the entire night and at 6:00AM received morphine, after which she finally slept. At this time, the nurse noted her vital signs, which was again part of the routine preparation for fever treatment. While we do not have the fever chart record, we do have the clinical chart from the ward to which she returned after the end of her treatment around 5:00 PM. It was noted that she was talkative but "well taken", but her vital signs betrayed that she was close to shock. It would be an exaggeration to describe her condition as "good". The terms that nurses used to describe the conditions of their patients were often not meaningful – terms such as fair, good, treatment well taken, pulse good/poor quality, etc. However, the main concern of the nurses seemed to be Connie B's behaviour; she was so "restless and talkative", she received Morphine by injection. Connie B. was seen by psychiatrists several times (the blood pressure was taken by a physician) and after the first injection, it was reported that she "sleeps from 11–4am. Very disturbed on awakening. Out of bed". Again the nurses classified this disturbed behaviour as something that had to be corrected and not something that was the result of the treatment (and the interventions endured during the weeks before treatment). The nurses only registered that Connie B. was "out of the bed", which was against regulations, and described her as "impulsive" (4:10AM). As a consequence, she received another Morphine injection at 4:30AM and the nurse noted afterwards that she was "quieter, sleeping". At 9:30AM, Connie B. was transferred to the regular ward. No daily notes exist from 16 December but a protocol inserted in the chart suggests that she received another three-hour pack during the night and a morphine injection at 12:30 AM. She was still described as "talkative + noisy. Singing. Crying + noisy" (Pack, Dec. 16–39, 12:30–1:30). From 1:45AM on, the nurse noted that Connie B. slept and summarized at 3:00AM "Pulse good volume. Removed from CWP [since she] Slept 1 ½ hours in pack after hypo [which is the abbreviation for injection]".

Connie B.'s death

Her treatment into January remained the same, where she commuted between bath, pack and ward. On 2 January her "Condition [was] much the same shouting singing + yelling very excited. One day appetite very good – the next thinks food is poisoned + has to be tube fed. Unclean + self abusive" (Reports Dec. 39). However, on 5 Jan 1940, the nurse noted that she had "suffered a weak spell last night [.] today appears to be exhausted but is so un-co-operative + unreasonable [-] unable to persuade Pt. to remain in bed – given sedative". The description "weak spell" is an understatement. According to the bath reports, Connie B. had spent most of the afternoon and evening in a continuous bath. That night, she appeared "exhausted. Removed from CWP immediately. Pulse rapid and poor. Resp[iration] rapid + shallow. 12:50AM Dr. Randall notified". At 1:05AM, the nurse noted that "Coramine 1 amp:

Intravenously by Dr. Randall. Resp[iration] and colour slightly improved" but 5 minutes later, Connie received another intravenous injection of Cormanine and 3amp. Digafoline intramuscularly. The nurse noted "pulse improving. Alcohol sponge" (1:10AM). No pulse nor repiration was noted and at 1:30AM the body temperature was 105 degrees F. At 1:45 Connie got another injection of Coramine and the "cold sponge continued". The nurse noted "Last rights administered by Priest. Colour, pulse much improved. Visited by relatives". The nurses and psychiatrist obviously concluded that Connie would not survive the night and at 2:45 AM she received an injection of Morphium Sulphate and again an injection of Digafoline. At 3:15 AM the nurse noted "Trembling through entire body". But even in this life-threatening situation, the nurse seemed to be mainly concerned with Connie's behaviour because at 3:30AM she noted "Fairly quiet. Trembling the entire body" and 15minutes later again reiterated that she was quiet even though vomiting a small amount. From this moment on, the nurses resumed their routine note-taking, recording her pulse and concentrating on her behaviour. At 6:00AM she was "sleeping at intervals. Pulse good quality. Resting quietly".

This incident demonstrates that Connie B.'s treatment was literally a life-threatening one. She had survived only by chance – if she had died during the night, her death would certainly not have been connected to the treatment that she received. The nurses' notes suggest that this incident possessed little significance for them and even though she had nearly died, the nurses concentrated on correcting Connie B's behaviour. On 5 January 1940 at 8:00AM her pulse was "fair volume, reg[ular] in force and frequency". Although she did not feel well and was vomiting, she became excited and "Very resistive, biting, scratching, + punching when out of bed". She was "returned to bed with difficulty" and received a sedative, and was tube fed water and orange juice. Her continuous baths resumed only three days after her near death.

Conclusion

In our opinion, nursing notes are a unique source not often used in in the history of psychiatry. Their examination provides a better understanding of the kind of treatment endured by patients in this Fever Unit, as well as of the relationships between nurses and patients. These notes reveal how specific treatments were used in everyday psychiatric practice. We argue that an analysis focusing merely on the texts left by psychiatrists in scientific articles, textbooks or even in the medical records, do not shed light on actual asylum practices. Based on our reading of these patient records, our findings contradict Bromley's assumption that complications of this treatment for neurosyphillis were of a minor nature, and merely caused discomfort to patients. Life-threatening events were an integral part of the patient experience. We have documented similar findings in all the patient files that we examined.

These nursing notes are particularly rich given that the nurses were solely responsible for the Fever Unit and patient treatment at the Ontario Hospital in Toronto. Our analysis of these nursing notes is preliminary, yet we believe that nurses appeared to be more concerned with patient behaviour than with the consequences of any life-threatening incidents. Patients obviously suffered and underwent multiple "small deaths" during their treatments. However, we do not notice any great empathy with patients or any concern for their welfare. We conclude our analysis with two preliminary hypotheses:

First, fever treatments were as much a means to discipline patients as they were to "cure" their physical ailments. This aspect is reinforced by the fact that in the 1940s some of the patients received shock treatments simultaneously to their fever treatment because they were considered unco-operative.

Second, nurses perceived their patients in the Fever Unit as somewhat less than human – and rather like, as we have argued elsewhere, as having lives unworthy of living. Further research into psychiatric practice will help us understand if these patterns still persist.

Bibliography

Archival sources

Archives of Ontario

Bernado A.: patient record number 25870. RG 10-278 Queen Street Mental Health Centre Fever Therapy Unit records: Boxes 1–4.

Bromley, A.J.: Letter to the Minister of Health & Report on the Treatment of Neurosphilis with Special Reference to Artificial Therapy (Registry: RG 10-20-B-9-454 (RG 10-278 Queen Street Mental Health Centre Fever Therapy Unit Box: B431584), box #4 ed.), 1939a.

Bromley, A.J.: Report on the treatment of neurosyphilis, with special reference to the use of artificial fever therapy at certain institution in the states of Michigan and Illinois, USA (Registry: RG 10-20-B-9-454 (RG 10-278 Queen Street Mental Health Centre Fever Therapy Unit Box: B431584, box 4 ed.), 1939b.

Bromley, A.J.: Artificial Fever in the Treatment of Neurosphyllis [Printed synopsis about fever treatement for hosital internal use] (Letter to the Minister of Health & Report on the Treatment of Neurosyphillis with Special Reference to Artificial Fever Therapy Doc. Registry: RG 10-20-B-9-454 (RG 10-278 Queen Street Mental Health Centre Fever Therapy Unit Box: B431584), 4 ed.): Ontario Hospital, Toronto, 1940.

Carl H. patient record number 20649. RG 10-278 Queen Street Mental Health Centre Fever Therapy Unit records: Boxes 1–4.

David G. patient record number 25451. RG 10-278 Queen Street Mental Health Centre Fever Therapy Unit records: Boxes 1–4.

Enrico C. patient record number 25760. RG 10-278 Queen Street Mental Health Centre Fever Therapy Unit records: Boxes 1–4.

Fever Unit Treatments (monthly). (1943–1954). Treatment lists (RG 10-278 Queen Street Mental Health Centre Fever Therapy Unit records, box 4, 462 ed.).

List of Neurosyphilitis Patients who are discharged or on probation following treatment and are adjusting satisfactorily. RG 10-20-B-9-463. RG 10-278 Queen Street Mental Health Centre Fever Therapy Unit records, box #4; 1941.

No author: Suggested List of equipment for Fever Therapy Clinic (RG 10-20-B-9-460 (RG 10-278 Queen Street Mental Health Centre Fever Therapy Unit Box: B431584), box #4 ed.), 1940.

Peter M. patient record [two records with different casebook numbers: 23249 and 23671]. RG 10-278 Queen Street Mental Health Centre Fever Therapy Unit records: Boxes 1–4.

Stephen O. patient record number 26599. RG 10-278 Queen Street Mental Health Centre Fever Therapy Unit records: Boxes 1–4.

Unsuitable cases. RG 10-278 Queen Street Mental Health Centre Fever Therapy Unit records, box #4; 1940.

William W. patient record number 23002. RG 10-278 Queen Street Mental Health Centre Fever Therapy Unit records: Boxes 1–4.

Printed sources

Barcroft, Joseph: On Anoxæmia. In: The Lancet 196 (1920), p. 489. doi:http://dx.doi.org/10.1016/S0140-6736(00)54692-3.

Belt, Elmer; Folkenberg, Alvin W.: Gonorrhea: it's treatment by artificial fever, and by fever therapy in combination with sulfanamide. In: California and Western Medicine 52 (1940), 4, p. 172.

Bromberg, Leon: Artificial Fever Therapy. In: The American Journal of Nursing 36 (1936), 12, pp. 1183–1190. doi:10.2307/3414256.

Brown, Herbert R.; Clark, William F.; Jones, Nathaniel; Walther, Johanna; Warren, Stafford L.: The Relationship of Dehydration and Overhydration of the Blood Plasma to Collapse in the Management of Artificial Fever Therapy. In: Journal of Clinical Investigation 22 (1943), 4, p. 485.

Brown, Wade H; Pearce, Louise: Tryparsamide: It's action and use. In: Journal of the American Medical Association 82 (1924), 1, p. 9.

Cole, H. N.; Driver. J. R.; Hutton, J. G.: Mercurosal in the Treatment of Syphilis. In: The Journal of the American Medical Association 79 (1922), 22, p. 1824.

Courville, Cyril B.: Asphyxia as a Consequence of Nitrous Oxide Anesthesia. In: Medicine 15 (1936), p. 247.

Crawford, C. M.: Paretic Neurosyphilis. History, Pathogenesis, Neuropathology, Treatment. In: The Ontario Journal of Neuro-Psychiatry (1921), pp. 25–32.

Ebaugh, Franklin. G., & Dickson, Rogers. W.: The Use of Tryparsamide in the Treatment of General Paralysis: Results of the First Year's Experience. In: The Journal of the American Medical Association 83 (1924), 11, 807.

Gore, Ira; Isaacson, Norman: The Pathology of Hyperpyrexia; Observations at Autopsy in 17 Cases of Fever Therapy. In: American journal of Pathology 25 (1949), 5, p. 1059.

Harrison, Lawrence. W.: Modern Diagnosis and Treatment of Syphilis, Chancroid and Gonorrhoea. Toronto 1925.

Hartman, F. W.: Lesions of the Brain Following Fever Therapy. In: Journal of the American Medical Association, 109 (1937), 26, p. 2121. doi:10.1001/jama.1937.02780520006002.

Hicks, Myers H.; Holt, Howard P.; Guerrant, John L.; Leavell, Byrd S.: (1948). The Effect of Spontaneous and Artificially induced Fever on Liver Function. In: Journal of Clinical Investigation 27 (1948), 5, p. 587.

Hospital Division Department of Health: 76th Annual Report of the Hospital Division Department of Health upon the Ontario Hospitals for the Mentally Ill, Mentally Defective,

Epileptic and Habituate Patients of the Province of Ontarion for the Year Ending March 31st, 1943. Toronto, 1944.

Hospital Division Department of Mental Health: 64th Annual Report of the Hospital Division Department of Health upon the Ontario Hospitals for the Mentally Ill, Mentally Subnormal and Epileptic of the Province of Ontarion for the Year which ended 31st October 1931 The Legislative Assembly of Ontario, Sessional Paper N0. 15, 1932 (Microfilm B117 Reel 1, Ontario Dept. of Health. reports upon Ontario Mental Hsopitals & Mental Health Services 1931 to 1941 ed.). Toronto, 1932.

Hospital Division Department of Mental Health: 66th Annual Report of the Hospital Division Department of Health upon the Ontario Hospitals for the Mentally Ill, Mentally Defective, Epileptic and Habituate Patients of the Province of Ontario for the Year Ending October 31st, 1933 (Microfilm B117 Reel 1, Ontario Dept. of Health. reports upon Ontario Mental Hospitals & Mental Health Services 1931 to 1941 ed.). Toronto, 1934.

Hospital Division Department of Mental Health: 70th Annual Report of the Hospital Division Department of Health upon the Ontario Hospitals for the Mentally Ill, Mentally Defective, Epileptic and Habituate Patients of the Province of Ontario for the Year Ending March 31st, 1937 (Microfilm B117 Reel 1 Ontario Dept. of Health. reports upon Ontario Mental Hospitals & Mental Health Services 1931 to 1941 ed.). Toronto, 1938.

Hospital Division Department of Mental Health: 73rd Annual Report of the Hospital Division Department of Health upon the Ontario Hospitals for the Mentally Ill, Mentally Defective, Epileptic and Habituate Patients of the Province of Ontario for the Year Ending March 31st, 1940 (Microfilm B117 Reel 1 – Ontario Dept. of Health. reports upon Ontario Mental Hsopitals & Mental Health Services 1931 to 1941 ed.) Toronto, 1941.

Hospitals Division Department of Health: 83rd Annual Report of the Hospital Division Department of Health upon the Ontario Hospitals for the Mentally Ill, Mentally Defective, Epileptic and Habituate Patients of the Province of Ontario Calendar Year 1949. Toronto, 1950.

Kruif, Paul de: Machine Fever. In: Country Gentleman, April 1937, pp. 7–8, 40, 43, 45–46.

Kruif, Paul de: Found: A One-Day Cure for Syphilis. In: Reader's Digest, September 1942, pp. 10–14.

Kruif, Paul de: Stamping Out Syphilis with the One-Day Treatment. Reader's Digest, December 1943, pp. 105–108.

Landis, Eugene. M.: Micro-Injection studies of Capillary Permeability. III. The Effect of Lack of Oxygen on the Permeability of the Capillary Wall to Fluid and to the Plasma Proteins. In: American Journal of Physiology 83 (1928), January, pp. 528–542.

Lehmann, Emmy: Nursing Care in Fever Treatment. In: The American Journal of Nursing 37 (1937), 12, pp. 1315–1321.

Lutz, Francis. M.: Nursing Care in Artificial Fever Therapy. In: The American Journal of Nursing 36 (1936), 12, pp. 1191–1194.

Malcolm, Mabel M.: Non-Typical Wassermanns in Spinal Fluids. In: The Public Health Journal 18 (1927), 3, pp. 115–117.

McKay, Hugh A.; Gray, Kenneth G.; Winans, William C. (1933). Diathermy in treatment of general paresis. In: The Ontario Journal of Neuro-Psychiatry (March 1933), pp. 53–61.

McKay, Hugh A.; Winans, William C.: Diathermy in treatment of general paresis. In: American Journal of Psychiatry 82 (1932), 3, pp. 531–539.

Peterson, S. C.: The Use of Marphasen in the Treatment of Syphilis. In: The Canadian Medical Association Journal (Februray 1937), pp. 172–173.

Pollock, Hoartio M.: The Economic Loss to the State of New York on Account of Syphilitic Mental Diseases During the Fiscal Year Ending June 30, 1917. In: Mental Hygiene 2 (1918), pp. 277–282.

Pollock, Hoartio M.: Economic Loss on Account of Hospital Cases of Mental Disease and Associated Physical Disorders in New York State, 1928. In: Psychiatric Quaterly 3 (1929), pp. 186–195.

Schaffle, Karl; Riesenberg, Max: The Occurence of Positive Wassermann Reactions in the Spinal Fluid of Tuberculous and Other Nonsyphilitic Cases of Meningitis. In: American Journal of Medical Science 178 (1929), 623–637.

Scott, Virgil; Reynolds, F. W.: Biologic False Positive Spinal Fluid Wassermann Reactions Associated with Meningitis: Report of Eight Cases. In: American Journal of Syphilis, Gonorrhea and Venereal Diseases 19 (1944), n. p.

Simpson, Walter M.: Artificial Fever Therapy of Syphilis. In: Journal of the American Medical Association 105 (1935), 26, pp. 2132–2140. doi:10.1001/jama.1935.02760520012003.

Telfer, G. W.: The Treatment of general Paresis by Diathermy. In: The Ontario Journal of Neuro-Psychiatry, September 1934, n. p.

Thompson, Loyd: Syphilis. New York 1920.

Secondary research literature

Borke, Jesse: Shock. In: MedlinePlus. Trusted Health Information for You (2015). Retrieved from https://www.nlm.nih.gov/medlineplus/ency/article/000039.htm, July 08, 2016.

Brandt, Allen M.: The Syphilis Epidemic and its Relation to AIDS. In: Science 239 (1988), 4838, p. 380.

Brown, William Jordan: Syphilis and Other Venereal Diseases. Massachusetts; Cambridge 1970.

Dowshen, Steven: Metabolism. TeensHealth from Nemours. June 2015. Retrieved from http://kidshealth.org/en/teens/metabolism.html, July 08, 2016.

Eghigian, G. (ed.): From Madness to Mental Health: Psychiatric Disorder and Its Treatment in Western civilization. New Brunswick/NJ 2010.

Fleck, Ludwik: Entstehung und Entwicklung einer wissenschaftlichen Tatsache. Einführung in die Lehre vom Denkstil und Denkkollektiv. Frankfurt/Main 1980.

Foth, Thomas: Nurses, Medical Records and the Killing of Sick Persons before, during and after the Nazi Regime in Germany. In: Nursing Inquiry 20 (2012), 2, pp. 93–100. doi:10.1111/j.1440-1800.2012.00596.x.

Hadjiliadis, Denis: Respiratory Alkalosis. In: MedlinePlus. Trusted Health Information for You (August 25, 2014). Retrieved from https://www.nlm.nih.gov/medlineplus/ency/article/000111.htm, July 08, 2016.

Hadjiliadis, Denis: Skin Discoloration – Bluish. In: MedlinePlus. Trusted Health Information for You (June 22, 2015). Retrieved from https://www.nlm.nih.gov/medlineplus/ency/article/000039.htm, July 08, 2016.

Higdon, Jane: Sodium (Chloride). In: Micronutrient Information Center (2001, November 2008 [Obazanek, Eva]). Retrieved from http://lpi.oregonstate.edu/mic/minerals/sodium, July 08, 2016.

Larrañaga de, Gabriela; Trombetta, Luis; Wingeyer, Silva P.; Remondino, Graciela: False Positive Reactions in Confirmatory Tests for Syphilis in Presence of Atiphospholipid Antibodies: Misdiagnosis with Prognostic and Social Consequences. In: Dermatology Online Journal 12 (2006), 4, p. 22.

Martin, Laura J.: Alkalosis. In: MedlinePlus. Trusted Health Information for You (2015, August 25, 2014). Retrieved from https://www.nlm.nih.gov/medlineplus/ency/article/000111.htm, July 08, 2016.

MedicineNet: Definition of Tetany. In: MedTerms Dictionary (2016, May 13, 2016). Retrieved from http://www.medicinenet.com/script/main/art.asp?articlekey=13312, July 08, 2016.

National Institute of Neurological Disorders and Stroke: Anoxia and Hypoxia. In: CNS Centre For Neuro Skills (n. y.). Retrieved from https://www.neuroskills.com/brain-injury/anoxia-and-hypoxia.php, July 08, 2016.

Patterson, Diana; Vilensky, Joel A.; Robertson, Wendy M.; Berger, Joseph: Treatment and Diagnostic Accuracy of Neurosyphilis at Boston City Hospital's Neurological Unit, 1930–1979. In: Journal of the Neurological Sciences 314 (2012), 1–2, pp. 1–4. doi:http://dx.doi.org/10.1016/j.jns.2011.11.007.

Tipliski, Veryl M.: Parting at the Crossroads: The Emergence of Education for Psychaitric Nursing in Three Canadian Provinces, 1909–1955. In: Canadian Bulletin of Medical History / Bulletin canadien d'histoire de la médecine 21 (2004), 2, pp. 253–279.

Verhave, Jan P.: Paul de Kruif, American science writer on malaria: a case study. In: MalariaWorld Journal 2 (2011), 1, pp. 1–6.

Young, Mary de: Encyclopedia of Asylum Therapeutics, 1750–1950s. Jefferson 2015.

Reform and Training of Psychiatric Nurses

"Fundamentally changed Duties" – The Introduction of Advanced Training for Nurses at the Psychiatric University Hospital Heidelberg as Part of the Early Psychiatric Reform in West Germany

Maike Rotzoll

Summary

Before psychiatric care was redesigned in the Federal Republic of Germany by the Enquete Commission of the German Bundestag and the Psychiatric Reform of the 1970s, there already was an ongoing process of change providing new stimuli for mental health services, which the historians Franz-Werner Kersting and Hans-Walter Schmuhl have called "reform before the reform".

The Psychiatric University Hospital of Heidelberg is a prominent example of these early reform aspirations. Here, Walter von Baeyer (1904–1987), who had held the Chair for Psychiatry since 1955, supported the social psychiatric activities of his two senior physicians, Karl Peter Kisker (1926–1997) and Heinz Häfner (*1926). Following the American concept of Community Mental Health Centers, a complete community-based psychiatric unit was introduced between 1960 and 1968, including transitional care institutions, outpatient care, industrial work therapy units and patients' clubs. Until Kisker went to Hannover in 1966, both protagonists led these projects together. From the very beginning, the reform of psychiatric nursing was regarded as a substantial part of any further progress in reform, which can also be seen in the introduction of participatory observation in one of the wards in 1965.

From no later than 1962, there were plans to establish advanced psychiatric nursing training. Its launch in 1963 was considered a milestone and one of the first essential steps on the path of the social psychiatric department to a "model unit". Whereas the establishment of advanced training is known, there has hardly been any research into the actual curriculum, the practical experiences of the participants and their professional development, interactions with patients or professionalization strategies and their effects on the later psychiatric reform. This contribution is intended to provide a beginning to remedy this deficiency in research.

Introduction: The "Department for Social Psychiatry and Rehabilitation" at the Psychiatric University Clinic Heidelberg[1]

In October 1963, the University of Munich initiated a survey of other universities. A psychiatric day-and-night clinic had just been established in Munich one year before. The survey was intended to see whether other places in Germany had implemented this advanced therapeutic conception of psychiatric

---

1   This text was partly written for research carried out by the author and entrusted to her by the "Verein zur Förderung der Stiftung Zentralinstitut für Seelische Gesundheit e. V." [Association for the Furtherance of the Foundation Central Institute for Mental Health], investigating the history of the Zentralinstitut für Seelische Gesundheit in Mannheim (opened in 1975). Cf. Häfner/Martini (2011).

transitional care institutions.[2] From the survey results it appears the University of Frankfurt and the University of Heidelberg had been trailblazers in this field.[3] In May 1959, the Frankfurt Psychiatric Clinic had "three night-clinic beds on a continual basis".[4] From this modest beginning, particularly since the adoption of the day-clinic treatments, they had developed a considerable range of options by 1963.[5] At this point in time, Frankfurt operated a patient club and a specialized outpatient clinic alongside the night- and day clinics (transitional care institutions) and two open wards. The social psychiatric institution was in charge of about 65 patients.[6]

Frankfurt became a model for the psychiatrists who led the pioneering social-psychiatric work at the Heidelberg hospital, beginning in 1960.[7] Supported by the hospital director Walter von Baeyer (1904–1987), two young senior physicians initiated essential steps from about 1958. Karl-Peter Kisker (1926–1997) had completed his clinical education in Heidelberg and moved to Hannover in 1966, and his colleague Heinz Häfner (*1926)[8] arrived from Munich in 1958.

In 1962, Kisker established the night clinic as the first transitional care institution in Heidelberg. The night clinic was preceded in 1960 by the creation of two rehabilitation wards as new extensions of the psychiatric clinic's "Garden Houses". Together they formed the preliminary stages of the later

2   Heidelberg, University Archive (UAH), Rep. 49/367, operation of the Psychiatric and Neurological Clinic. Day- and Night-Clinic 1962–68, letter from the administrative committee of the University of Munich dated 1/10/1963.

3   Loc. cit., letter from the administrative committee of the University of Munich dated 25.11.1963. In this letter it is reported that 103 in-patients and 47 out-patiens were treated in Frankfurt in the year 1962, and in Heidelberg a night-clinic exists, where 12 patients were "processed" in the same year. The information with regard to this is from the administration of the Clinical University Institutions and is dated 22/10/1963.

4   Kulenkampff (1961), p. 218.

5   UAH, Rep. 49/367, leaflet on the Frankfurt day clinic, sent as information to the Heidelberg administration of the Clinical University Institutions on 24/8/1962. The day clinic had been opened in April 1962.

6   Bosch (1967), p. 65; Cf. Rave-Schwank (1971).

7   Thus, an application made in August 1962 for "the experimental set-up of a night clinic with 2 additional beds in the cellar of the male pavilion section" refers expressly to the experience gathered in this kind of treatment in Frankfurt. UAH, Rep. 49/367, letter from Kisker to the administration of the Clinical University Institutes, dated 15/8/1962. The Director of Administration Ernst then inquired on 20/8/1962 of the University Clinic Frankfurt what nursing costs had been agreed on there. In a reply dated 24/8/1962 he received the information that the patients in the night clinic basically paid for themselves. This model was at first introduced at Heidelberg, too.

8   On Häfner's biography, cf. Sheperd (1982), pp. 42–44. Cf. further the article by Asmus Finzen on the occasion of Häfner's 60th birthday, entitled "Vorkämpfer der Sozialpsychiatrie" [Pioneer of Social Psychiatry] in the Frankfurter Allgemeine Zeitung of 20/5/1986, p. 27, and the article in the same newspaper by Rainer Flöhl, "Reformer am Wendepunkt" [Reformer at the Crossroads], on the occasion of Häfner's 70th birthday (20/5/1996, p. 33).

social psychiatry department.[9] According to the traditional gender segregation of the psychiatric clinic, there was a division in the rehabilitation ward between the pavilion for male patients (right wing of the building, Kisker) and the pavilion for female patients (left wing, Häfner). Both wards employed modern therapeutic experiences in terms of a "therapeutic community", aiming to reintegrate patients into society through rehabilitative treatment. Both rehabilitation wards had twelve beds at their disposal, since therapeutic groups consisting of twelve patients were deemed reasonable. The socio-therapeutic approach was supplemented by the use of psychoanalytic therapy groups and individual psychotherapy in an environment with as minimal a hierarchy as possible.[10]

In December 1963, Häfner applied to the Ministry of Cultural Affairs for the official establishment of a psychiatric rehabilitation department at the Heidelberg Clinic. Häfner strove for an independent social-psychiatric institution – primarily for research, and secondarily as a treatment facility. The department was officially established in Heidelberg in early 1965. Initially small, it served as the nucleus for the Central Institute for Mental Health in Mannheim, established in 1975, and as a kind of trendsetter for the Psychiatric Reform.[11] With the opening of the Day Clinic in 1967 (situated in some distance from the psychiatric clinic near Heidelberg Castle), the department represented a complete CMHC, a "Community Mental Health Center," after the U.S. model. No longer a large secluded institution, but at least partly in the heart of society, the department offered a set of possibilities for inpatient and outpatient treatment, in addition to the modern "semi-residential" transitional care institutions.[12]

9   Mannheim, Archive of the Central Institute for Mental Health (AZI), Häfner's application for an expertise from the science council on the planned model institute, dated 1/6/67. The annexes to the existing buildings were at first intended for insulin treatment and were finished towards the end of 1959. But soon von Baeyer agreed to the plan to offer modern social psychiatric services in the new rooms. UAH, Rep. 49/288, Administration of the Clinical University Institutes, Budget 1960. Here can be found the correspondence on the plans for the use of the annexes. Cf. also Häfner (1979), p. 155.

10 Cf. Häfner/Zerssen (1964); Häfner/Vogt-Heyder/Zerssen (1965); Häfner (1965). In 1965 the two clinics in the department were conjoined under Häfner's direction.

11 At this time, the "Abteilung für Sozialpsychiatrie und Rehabilitation" [Department for Social Psychiatry and Rehabilitation] consisted of the two clinical wards with their night-clinic beds in the cellar and therapeutic activities for discharged patients, such as post-clinical care and a therapeutic club. After the position of a "head of department" had been created from the 1/1/1965, Häfner had been named head of the Department in April. Cf. Häfner's letter to the member of state parliament, Karl Hauff, dated 18/11/1965, AZI, file on the model institute, Mannheim A-M 1964–66.

12 The core of the department was formed at this time by the two rehabilitation wards (still quartered in the small garden houses that actually belonged to the "main" psychiatric clinic), which offered ergotherapeutic and occupational therapy services, as well as night-clinic beds. In addition, there was further training in social psychiatry, post-discharge care, group and laymens' work, the halfway house in Rohrbach in Heidelberg, the day-clinic on the Schlossberg in the same town, and the research center for social psychiatric epidemiology. Cf. Rotzoll (2012).

The CMHC was a U.S. import. The desire to achieve international – western – standards played an important role in the reform movement ("reform before the reform").[13] The "westernization" in the politics of the psychiatric field reflected the general political tendencies of the time.[14] In February 1963, President John F. Kennedy (1917–1963) had delivered a message to the Congress entitled "Mental Illness and Mental Retardation", and it was his charisma that gave a special importance to the topic and a unique significance to his message.[15] In an international advanced training conference in Heidelberg, the Frankfurt professor of psychiatry, Jürg Zutt (1893–1980), expressed it in this way (his article was later published in the journal *Moderne Krankenpflege* ("Modern Nursing"): "President Kennedy's exemplary message to the United States Congress on the problem of mental health gives us the courage to believe that the same vigor seen in other parts of the world can inspire similar results here as well."[16]

"Greater, weightier tasks and more responsibility than ever before." The beginning of advanced social psychiatry training for nurses in Heidelberg

In order to make the urgency of the reforms clear and set the proposed Heidelberg department in a wider context, Häfner likewise referred to Kennedy's message in his application that very same year, 1963.[17] In addition, Häfner in his application pointed to a Heidelberg particularity: Häfner had established the first two-year advanced social psychiatric training program for nurses, as a pilot project beginning April 1, 1963. The goal was to prepare "suitable personnel for fundamentally changed duties" in the psychiatric ward.[18] The early implementation of advanced training for nurses was conducted from Häfner's "small, modern female ward."[19] This shows how central the mentality shift in nursing care appeared to him for the transition from a custodial model to an actively therapeutic psychiatric ward: it seemed to be very much a matter of

13 Hanrath (2002), p. 330–331.
14 The scientific operations in the Federal Republic oriented themselves towards that in Western countries early on; this process of integration was furthered by the escalation of the "cold war". Cf. Doering-Manteuffel (1999), pp. 68–70.
15 UAH, literary estate of Walter von Baeyer, Rep. 63/82, Report on the session of the Frankfurt Action Committee dated 25/6/1964 and a report on the session of the Action Committee dated 29/10/1964, as well as a German translation of the "special message" (17-page typescript on the structure of the community centers, cf. p. 6). On the Kennedy speech and its influence, cf. also Hanrath (2002), p. 333.
16 Zutt (1965), p. 5. Cf. auch v. Baeyer (1966).
17 UAH, Rep. 49/373. The five-page application, dated 12/12/1963, has von Baeyer's signature, but it was composed by Häfner, as shown by the dictation sign HH.
18 UAH, Rep. 49/373, application of 12/12/1963, p. 2.
19 At least since 1962 preparations had been in progress. This is shown by Häfner's request to the administration to announce the training program in corresponding journals, a request dated 25/9/1962, UAH, Rep. 49/293, summary of the budget plan for 1964.

"fruitful collaboration in the therapeutic community."[20] Without an appropriate education, in Häfner's opinion, the nurses could not withstand "this exceedingly difficult situation, being exposed to the emotional tensions and pathological demands of a group of patients" rather than facing it helplessly – in this way he described the experience in Heidelberg during the socio-therapeutic reorganization of the ward.[21] Häfner thus depicted the introduction of the advanced training of nurses as a productive response to distinct local experiences and insights.[22] In 1965, as confirmation for this view of the role of "traditional" nurses and for the necessity of a shift in mentality, came a "concealed participatory observation" pursued in the "garden house for male patients" of the Heidelberg Clinic and published later under the title, "The Masters of the Clinic". The results indicated that traditional nurses would seldom support modern therapeutic measures.[23]

The practical part of the advanced training was fulfilled by the nurses working continuously in the social psychiatry department. The theoretical part ran at the same time over the course of four semesters. The training programs from 1967 and 1971 are known. They consisted of both traditional issues (clinical psychiatry with case reviews and general psychopathology) and special social-psychiatric topics and aspects of group dynamics. As early as 1967, an introduction to child and youth psychiatry was added to the curriculum and this was continued. The program of 1971 was formulated more concretely and contained more practical exercises, such as role-playing.[24] A midterm and final exam were also provided.

---

20 Cf. Häfner (1974/1975), pp. 5–6 and pp. 10–12.
21 Häfner was of the opinion that the regular nursing training did not adequately prepare nurses for psychiatry. The introcuction of additional training took place at a time when nursing training was being discussed and re-ordered: in 1957 a two-year training period was left in the nursing law, but a third was added by way of practical training; in 1965 the period of training was established at three years and the number of hours of instruction considerably increased. Cf. Müller (2006), p. 3–16, here p. 13.
22 Cf. also Häfner/Zerssen (1964), p. 246. Kisker organized a corresponding program in Hanover after he moved there in 1966. Cf. Häfner (2003), p. 128 and the contribution by Christof Beyer in this book.
23 Hemprich/Kisker (1968). On this aspect of change in social psychiatry, cf. also Flegel (1966), pp. 161–163. The central significance attributed to social psychiatric training and further training for different professional groups is shown by Häfner's application directed at the Science Council and dated 1/6/1967 (Häfner's private papers), pp. 19–22. This reports that a Director of Education is allegedly usual at the big universities in the US. Subsequently, the various planned training programs for different professional groups are described, mostly distinguishing longer training programs and shorter further training programs. A relatively independent training director with his own department for the coordination of the manifold training programs for physicians, psychologists, social workers and nursing personnel was now a goal for the social psychiatric institution yet to be founded (Central Institute for Mental Health).
24 Sozialpsychiatrische Informationen [Journal Social Psychiatric Information], special number "Ausbildungs-Info" [Training Information] 1973, p. 41 and pp. 47–48. On role playing as part of the program: Rave-Schwank/Kallinke (1973).

After twelve years, the additional training program in social psychiatry for examinee nurses transferred to the "Central Institute for Mental Health" at Mannheim after its opening in 1975 – at that time the Heidelberg department for social psychiatry was integrated into the new institution. According to Häfner, the training would develop "in the Institute under substantially better teaching conditions than before".[25] After previous unsuccessful efforts to obtain state recognition, the German Hospital Society approved the program in 1973.[26] Official state recognition followed in March 1980.[27] In the meantime, an additional class on child and youth therapy had been established.[28] The advanced training was a success and is still running today. Häfner wrote in 1979 with satisfaction that 65% of the graduates had obtained leading positions in social psychiatric institutions. This was a goal he had aimed at, in order to disseminate the ideas most effectively.[29]

But back to the beginning: while Frankfurt can claim to have had the "oldest, largest and most structured" social psychiatry rehabilitation department, Heidelberg's advanced training program for nurses may be seen as the first of its kind in the BRD. In his anthology of programs, published in 1973, Gregor Bosch designated it as the "mother of several grown-up children".[30] There is no connection to earlier "nursing schools" in psychiatric mental hospitals,

---

25 Manuscript on modern psychiatric care by Reinhold Becker and Heinz Häfner, Mannheim, Stadtarchiv, Sammlung Quellen und Dokumente Martini (SQDM) [City Archives, Martini Sources and Documents Collection], Ordner [File] II.

26 Central Institute for Mental Health (ZI), biannual report 1980/81, p. 183. A part of the official recognition was formed by the desire for the graduates of the program to be given a higher pay rating, advocated by Häfner already in 1969. Cf. Häfner/Martini (2011), p. 31 and pp. 35–36. This succeeded in 1977. Already in the training programs of 1967 and 1971 it is stated that application has already been made for state recognition: Sozialpsychiatrische Informationen [Journal Social Psychiatric Information], special number "Ausbildungs-Info" [Training Information] 1973, p. 40 and p. 46.

27 To further cement the recognition of this training program, an application was made to the Ministry for Health in Stuttgart in the summer of 1979 for state recognition. On 11 März 1980 the further training institution was recognised by the state. Cf. Häfner/Martini (2011), p. 36.

28 ZI, biannual report 1978/79, pp. 56–57. In the course that started in April 1979 with 21 participants, thirteen of them chose the major "General Psychiatry" and eight the major "Child and Youth Psychiatry".

29 ZI, biannual report 1978/79, pp. 56–57.

30 Bosch (1973), p. 4. He writes that the "Kieler Jahreskurs" [Kiel Yearly Course] was supposedly the first additional training program in the FR Germany: "Es bezieht jedoch die Neurologie mit ein und wurde, wohl auch wegen seines konventionellen Zuschnitts in der angelaufenen Diskussion wenig beachtet. [However, he includes neurology, and was not paid much attention, probably also because of his conventional position in the running debate]" The Kiel program was described on pp. 27–37 of the special number, but there is no information on when this one-year program was first initiated. The Frankfurt Training Program of 1967, with the above-cited passage, is briefly characterized on pp. 49–50, but it was a two-year program. According to Häfner/Martini (2011), p. 35, Frankfurt and Tübingen were among the first, as were München-Haar and Regensburg, to take over the Heidelberg program.

such as existed in Baden during the Weimar Republic, to be found in the program or in publications on the advanced training.[31]

Its implementation, and the question of who had the idea, need to be examined more closely. In the narrative of Häfner and other protagonists from the field of reform-oriented Heidelberg psychiatry, the initiatives for the advanced training program are described as resulting from local difficulties with nurses during the installation of the rehabilitation wards. Consequently, the training course was mostly doctor-led: at first by Detlev v. Zerssen (*1926), who soon after transferred to Munich, then for a short time by the psychologist Wiltrud Ranabauer (later Häfner-Ranabauer), and from 1969 to 1974 by Maria Rave-Schwank (*1935), head of the Heidelberg day-clinic.[32] In an article on the history of the training course from 1973, she described the reason behind the difficulties more concretely:

> The set-up of the social psychiatric department at the Psychiatric University Clinic Heidelberg faced difficulties early on with the nuns then employed. They and also the lay nurses had difficulties with the mainly younger and intelligent schizophrenic patients, who expressed criticism and questioned their nursing authority. These difficulties – which are understandable considering the close contact with patients and the addition of new and diverse tasks for the nuns and nurses – led to the development of Heidelberg's advanced training program.[33]

Risk democracy? New goals and new roles

From a medical perspective, the difficulties were inherent in the very principle of a "therapeutic community," a concept introduced by the psychiatrist Maxwell Jones (1907–1990) in 1953.[34] In contrast to the conservative hospital system, which seemed to produce "passive-dependent and submissive behaviors" on the part of nurses, the system developing in Heidelberg strove for a "personally represented, democratized authority open to discussion".[35] The aim was for a "partnership between patients, nurses and doctors", who together would pursue "the objective of providing optimal help for their sick members", so that all medical procedures could be clarified and discussed. This was thought to bring about a "demythologization of the medical role and the power of nurse personnel", creating an atmosphere of openness and trust as a precondition for the active cooperation "of patients".[36]

---

31 Thus, from 1921 in the Illenau, and from 1922 in Wiesloch, there were "nursing schools" for a few years which were to ensure the quality of nursing and the rise to higher rates of pay. The two-year training period had practical and theoretical elements which were only partly specific to psychiatry. Cf. Janzowski (2015), pp. 50–53.

32 Maria Rave-Schwank was also the first Heidelberg psychiatrist after the war to intensively work with the now-famous Prinzhorn Collection.

33 Rave-Schwank (1973a). Cf. also Rave-Schwank (1973b).

34 Jones (1976).

35 Häfner/Vogt-Heyder/Zerssen (1965), p. 104.

36 Häfner/Vogt-Heyder/Zerssen (1965), pp. 104–105.

While no uncertainty about the new concept was attributed to the doctors in the above cited publication, a certain discomfiture is ascribed to the nurses of the ward for female patients (two nuns and two regular nurses) by the following statement:

> The main difficulties rested first in this, that the group discussions led to the insecurity of nurses who were used to having inviolable authority. It engendered anxious, mistrustful and aggressive reactions. [...] The attempt to take the nurses to the therapeutic groups together with the patients failed: the critique on the part of the patients seemed unbearable to the nurses, and they reproached the doctor for not protecting them enough. Secondly, the same difficulties emerged with the attempt to have the nurses not only promote the patients' autonomy, but also implement the treatment program. Most of the nurses found it impossible to hold active group meetings with the patients in the afternoons. The insecurity over customary roles led to anxiety and contentions between the nurses, tensions with the patients, and resentful jealousy towards the close therapeutic contact between patients and doctors."

In short, following this description, it came to a "chaotic reaction" and "psychotic crisis". It otherwise seemed to prove that typical nursing education promoted a kind of "motherly-authority designed to instill passive and regressive behavior in patients". These factors stimulated a resolution to recruit new nurses to mature and develop within the framework of a two-year social psychiatry program. Thus, seven young examinee nurses, mostly high school graduates – a factor worth emphasizing to the authors – began the program in 1963. However, they too displayed emotional insecurity. Since the ward meetings with the doctor had not been sufficient for the "stabilization of the nurse groups", it was determined that the senior physician would lead "a therapeutic encounter group for the nurses as well".[37]

It was apparent that the program's candidates found this problematic. Maria Rave-Schwank noted that these therapeutic groups centered on the nurses were replaced by Balint groups (groups for therapeutic personnel to speak about the patients and their relationship to the staff, not about personal problems – such groups were introduced by the British psychiatrist Michael Balint (1896–1970) beginning in the 1950s on the basis of psychoanalytic theories[38]) in a later version of the training program due to the candidates' understandable desire for some distance from their colleagues.[39] Regarding this development, Gregor Bosch commented that the program grew increasingly more pragmatic over the years, corresponding to the "transformation of the institu-

37 Häfner/Vogt-Heyder/Zerssen (1965), pp. 108–109.
38 Balint (1954).
39 Rave-Schwank (1973a), p. 43: "While in earlier training courses this discussion group was conceived of as being stronger than the self-experience group, now the discussion of professional conflicts and problems in the sense of a Balint group has come to the fore. In this way we have to some extent fulfilled the understandable wish of the course participants to enable distance among each other, as work colleagues; cf. the leaflet."

tion from a psychosis-therapeutic trial ward to a developing large social psychiatry institution".[40]

The training candidates prevailed in at least this one point – a move which actually aligned with the democratic intention of the program – against the authority and interpretive power of the doctors. But perhaps it is more the question of whether or not they connected their own professionalization strategy with the program – especially as the social psychiatry approach ascribed a more independent role to them. Another question is whether or not the training programs in the U.S.-American and British institutions – from which Heidelberg and the BRD derived their general model of social psychiatry – had an impact on the implementation of the advanced training program at Heidelberg.

In his famous message to Congress, Kennedy held – at least in general terms – that the implementation of the new mental health program required having trained people at disposal. Along with psychiatrists, clinical psychologists, and social workers, he mentioned the need for continuously well-trained nurses.[41] In a memorandum from 1965, right after his assertion that "the situation with non-medical personnel is catastrophic," Häfner cited American literature on the role of nurses in modern forms of treatment as having a "key socio-therapeutic position".[42]

In their book entitled "Psychiatric Nursing" (1974), Maria Rave-Schwank and Christa Winter-v. Lersner referred to an American textbook written by the nurse Dorothy Mereness.[43] Mereness had introduced proposals for the education of psychiatric nurses as early as 1956 in her dissertation at Columbia University entitled "The Influence of Interdisciplinary Planning and Coordination upon the Role and Education of the Psychiatric Nurse."[44]

Its own textbook, new strategies?

As mentioned, the advanced training program in Heidelberg was essentially shaped by academic hospital personnel. The preparation of the textbook re-

40 Bosch (1973), p. 4. Bosch regrets only being able to precede the program of 1971 with that of 1967 in his collection, as this makes the road taken in Heidelberg only partly visible. This road has led from a program completely determined and defined by psychoanalytic training in self-experience and that of others, "über Krisen und Zwischenstufen zu einem bescheideneren und praxisgerechteren Anspruch [through crises and intermediate stages to a more modest and better practical standard]".

41 UAH, literary estate of Walter von Baeyer, Rep. 63/82, translation of the Kennedy message for the Action Committee. After visiting the US, v. Baeyer, in his reprot on the trip of 1967, pp. 3–4, points out that the NIMH position also provided money for the training of psychiatric expert staff, "Schwestern, Sozialarbeitern, Rehablitation-Counselors, klinischen Psychologen [nurses, social workers, rehab counsellors, clinical psychologists]", UAH, literary estate of Walter von Baeyer, Rep. 63/88, trip report by von Baeyer.

42 Häfner/Baeyer/Kisker (1965); Stanton/Schwartz (1954); Belknap (1956).

43 Mereness/Karnosh (1966).

44 Anonym (1960), p. 102–103 (Short review).

sulted in the cooperation of Maria Rave-Schwank and the teaching nurse
Christa Winter-v. Lersner, who had completed a psychiatric training program.
Upon closer examination, however, it is apparent that Christa Winter-v. Lersner had written fewer, and to some extent more traditional, chapters (such as
on nursing tasks in physical examination and somatic therapeutic methods).
As the foreword states, the book was aimed explicitly at "nurses and care-tak-
ers". It addressed first of all the intended transformation of roles:

> You have often assumed the role of "custodian", of guard, from your predecessors. Your
> main duties still consist of monitoring and surveillance. But many of you wonder how
> this can be done better; many would want to participate in a treatment program as a
> therapist if they only knew how.[45]

The text goes on to say that the profession acquires a "great new significance".
Instead of mere supervision over patients, participation in real therapeutic
work was now in demand. However, this required a different mentality, an
open-minded mentality, especially important since the nursing group spent
entire 24-hour days with the patients – divided in shift work within the nursing staff of the ward. Respect and responsible handling of information was
stressed, along with the sensible distribution of tasks within the wards. It
seemed no longer acceptable to give the unpleasant responsibilities to the
patients – they should no longer be seen as the "lowest members of a hierarchical stepladder". Essentially, everything in the book can be summed up as
one main task: the "organization of a ward into a therapeutic milieu".[46] The
inner-ward hierarchy should no longer be evident; the highest-ranking offi-
cials cannot claim the privilege of hiding behind desk work, but rather must
provide a model of "being present", "being with the patients", communicating
and relaying information to the doctor. Alongside the formation of the ward's
environment to be as "normal" a milieu as possible, the text addresses the
influence of time management, the rules of life in the ward, responsibility for
the outward appearance of the patients, the formation of "activation groups",
and ward gatherings. The common forms of therapy, from occupational therapy to psychotherapy, are ascribed to other professional groups. But the book
also addresses the wide range of new, yet basic extramural psychiatric duties
associated with the role – such as the formation of patient clubs, work in both
day- and night-clinics, time spent on the phone, and home visits. These factors
highlight how elements of nursing can resemble the tasks of a social worker,
but in a more traditional medical field. Nurses, for example, had to regularly
monitor any potential neglect and the patients' intake of medication, tasks
categorized as "important responsibilities outside the hospital."[47]

If we look at this role description, it is no wonder that more women than
men took it on and became psychiatric nurses – besides the fact that more
men worked as male nurses in psychiatry than in other medical disciplines. In

45   Rave-Schwank / Winter-v. Lersner (1974), preface, p. V.
46   Rave-Schwank / Winter-v. Lersner (1974), p. 6.
47   Rave-Schwank / Winter-v. Lersner (1974), p. 138.

fact, a few years later, Maria Rave-Schwank believed that the prevalence of female nurses was one of the problems of modern psychiatric care, as it supposedly seemed bad for the image of psychiatric nursing. On the one hand, an approach using motherly authority appeared no longer desirable. On the other hand, the rather inconspicuous, pleasant climate aspired to in the ward, with a smooth, friendly flow of work as a basis for the "actual" therapy seemed to involve abilities and willingness to submission often ascribed to women. This also applied to child and youth psychiatry. In his textbook of 1979, Remschmidt ascribed two main tasks to nurses, "the co-creation of the ward's milieu (its therapeutic climate) and […] the take-over of more circumscribed tasks within the scope of a treatment plan".[48]

With all of the reform-mindedness, the textbooks ultimately imputed to nursing personnel a rather subordinate assistant role, providing support for other people's concepts, rather than their own distinct modernizing initiatives. It sounded almost like a comforting encouragement when Maria Rave-Schwank stated at the end of her book:

> Nurses and care-workers need to know that not only must they learn something new and transform their relationships with the patients, but likewise also the doctors. Some reform-minded nurses have already been restrained by doctors who wanted nothing to do with such "modern frippery".[49]

Conclusion

There is a narrative that the medical doctors implemented the advanced training program to put forward "their" reform, and it is proved by the sources that Häfner indeed initiated and implemented the program. Yet there were also existing western models of advanced training for psychiatric nurses and favoring a stronger, more independent role of the nurses, as Maria Rave-Schwank stated in an interview referring to Great Britain. She also insisted on an increasingly active role for nurses: at first many of them wanted to attend the new educational program, later on they played an ever more involved role in the reform process.

---

48   Remschmidt (1979), p. 387.
49   Rave-Schwank / Winter-v. Lersner, p. 153.

Bibliography

Archival sources

University Archive Heidelberg (UAH) Rep. 63/82 Literary estate of Walter von Baeyer.

Printed sources

Anonym: Short Review on Mereness, Dorothy: "The Influence of Interdisciplinary Planning and Coordination upon the Role and Education of the Psychiatric Nurse." In: Nursing Research 9 (1960), pp. 102–103.

Baeyer, Walter von: Die Zukunft der psychiatrischen Krankenversorgung. In: Deutsches Zentralblatt für Krankenpflege 11 (1966), pp. 488–490.

Michael Balint: Training General Practitioners in Psychotherapy. British Medical Journal 1 (1954), pp. 115–120.

Belknap, I.: Human Problems of a State Mental Hospital. New York; Toronto; London 1956.

Bosch, Gregor: Soziale Wiedereingliederung psychisch Kranker vom Standpunkt der Universitätskliniken. In: Deutscher Verein für öffentliche und private Fürsorge (ed.): Die Verantwortung der Gesellschaft für ihre psychisch Kranken. Bericht über die Hauptausschusstagung am 5. und 6. Mai 1966 in Kiel (Schriften des Deutschen Vereins für öffentliche und private Fürsorge Bd. 235). Frankfurt 1967, pp. 64–77.

Bosch, Gregor: Zur Einführung. In: Sozialpsychiatrische Informationen, Sonderheft "Ausbildungs-Info" (1973), pp. 2–8.

Flegel, Horst: Die psychiatrische Krankenabteilung als therapeutische Gemeinschaft. In: Der Nervenarzt 37 (1966), pp. 160–164.

Häfner, Heinz; von Zerssen, Detlev: Soziale Rehabilitation, ein integrierender Bestandteil psychiatrischer Therapie. In: Der Nervenarzt 35 (1964), pp. 242–247.

Häfner, Heinz: Über die Rehabilitation jugendlicher Schizophrener. In: Fortschritte der Medizin 83 (1965), S. 541–546.

Häfner, Heinz; Baeyer, Walter von; Kisker, Klaus Peter: Dringliche Reformen in der psychiatrischen Krankenversorgung der Bundesrepublik. Über die Notwendigkeit des Aufbaus sozialpsychiatrischer Einrichtungen (psychiatrischer Gemeindezentren). In: Helfen und Heilen – Diagnose und Therapie in der Rehabilitation, Heft 4, Sonderdruck (1965).

Häfner, Heinz; Vogt-Heyder, B.; von Zerssen, Detlev: Erfahrungen mit Schizophrenen in einem gleitenden klinischen Behandlungs- und Nachsorgesystem. In: Zeitschrift für Psychotherapie und medizinische Psychologie 15 (1965), pp. 97–116.

Häfner, Heinz: Sozialpsychiatrische Arbeit im Krankenhaus. Sonderdruck aus Ärztliche Praxis 26 (1974), Heft Nr. 100 und 27 (1975), Heft Nr. 9.

Hemprich, R. D.; Kisker, Karl-Peter: Die "Herren der Klinik" und die Patienten. Erfahrungen aus der teilnehmend-verdeckten Beobachtung einer psychiatrischen Station. In: Der Nervenarzt 39 (1968), pp. 433–441.

Jones, Maxwell: Prinzipien der therapeutischen Gemeinschaft: soziales Lernen um'nd Sozialpsychiatrie. Bern u. a. 1976.

Kulenkampff, Caspar: Über die psychiatrische Nachtklinik. In: Der Nervenarzt 32 (1961), pp. 217–222.

Mereness, Dorothy Karnosh; Louis, J.: Essentials of Psychiatric Nursing. St Louis 1966.

Rave-Schwank, Maria: Évolution de la clinique socio-psychiatrique de Heidelberg-Mannheim. Information Psychiatrique 47 (1971), pp. 343–347.

Rave-Schwank, Maria: Sozialpsychiatrische Fachausbildung für Schwestern und Pfleger an der Sozialpsychiatrischen Klinik Heidelberg-Mannheim II (1971). In: Sozialpsychiatrische Informationen, Sonderheft "Ausbildungs-Info" (1973a), pp. 42–48.

Rave-Schwank, Maria; Kallinke, Dieter: Das Rollenspiel in der Ausbildung von Schwestern und Pflegern. Einige lernpsychologische Aspekte. In: Gruppendynamik. Forschung und Praxis 4(1973), pp. 35–41.

Rave-Schwank, Maria: Sozialpsychiatrische Fachausbildung für Krankenschwestern und Krankenpfleger. In: Deutsche Krankenpflegezeitschrift 26 (1973b), pp. 11–13.

Rave-Schwank, Maria; Winter-v. Lersner, Christa: Psychiatrische Krankenpflege. Eine praktische Einführung für Schwestern und Pfleger. Stuttgart 1974.

Remschmidt, Helmut: Kinder- und Jugendpsychiatrie. Praktische Einführung für Krankenpflege, pädagogische und soziale Berufe. Stuttgart 1979.

Sozialpsychiatrische Informationen, Sonderheft "Ausbildungs-Info" 1973.

Stanton, Alfred H.; Schwartz, Morris S.: The Mental Hospital. A Study of Institutional Participation in Psychiatric Illness and Treatment. New York 1954.

Zutt, Jürg: Über die neuen Krankenhausformen. Vortrag, gehalten auf dem Internationalen Fortbildungskongreß in Heidelberg 1964 (Sonderdruck aus "Moderne Krankenpflege", Heft 1/1965).

Secondary research literature

Doering-Manteuffel, Anselm: Wie westlich sind die Deutschen? Amerikanisierung und Westernisierung im 20. Jahrhundert. Göttingen 1999.

Häfner, Heinz: Die Geschichte der Sozialpsychiatrie in Heidelberg. In: Janzarik, Werner (ed.), Psychopathologie als Grundlagenwissenschaft (Klinische Psychologie und Psychopathologie Bd. 8). Stuttgart 1979, pp. 145–160.

Häfner, Heinz: Die Inquisition der psychisch Kranken geht ihrem Ende entgegen. Die Geschichte der Psychiatrie-Enquete und Psychiatriereform in Deutschland. In: Kersting, Franz-Werner (ed.): Psychiatriereform als Gesellschaftsreform. Die Hypothek des Nationalsozialismus und der Aufbruch der sechziger Jahre (Forschungen zur Regionalgeschichte, Band 46). Paderborn; München; Wien; Zürich 2003, pp. 113–140.

Häfner, Heinz; Martini, Hans: Das Zentralinstitut für Seelische Gesundheit. Gründungsgeschichte und Gegenwart. München 2011.

Hanrath, Sabine: Zwischen "Euthanasie" und Psychiatriereform. Anstaltspsychiatrie in Westfalen und Brandenburg: Ein deutsch-deutscher Vergleich (Forschungen zur Regionalgeschichte, Band 41). Paderborn; München; Wien; Zürich 2002.

Janzowski, Frank: Die NS-Vergangenheit in der Heil- und Pflegeanstalt Wiesloch. "… so intensiv wenden wir unsere Arbeitskraft der Ausschaltung der Erbkranken zu". Ubstadt-Weiher 2015.

Müller, Thomas: Zur Geschichte der Psychiatrie und der psychiatrischen Krankenpflege im deutschsprachigen Raum. In: Gaßmann, Mirjam u.a. (ed.): Psychiatrische Gesundheits- und Krankenpflege. Heidelberg u.a. 2006, p. 3–16.

Rotzoll, Maike: Die Entstehung der "Sozialpsychiatrischen Klinik Heidelberg" in den 1960er Jahren. Sozialpsychiatrie in Heidelberg. In: Heidelberg. Jahrbuch zur Geschichte der Stadt 17 (2013), pp. 133–148.

Sheperd, Michael (ed.): Psychiatrists on Psychiatry. Cambridge; London u.a. 1982.

From Nurse to "Sociagouge"? Ambitions, Realisation and Practise of Social Psychiatric Training at Hanover Medical School against the Background of the German Psychiatric Reform

Christof Beyer

Summary

In the run-up of the psychiatric reforms in Federal Germany of the 1970s, initiators of institutional changes emphasised the key role of psychiatric nurses in the restructuring of therapy in terms of social psychiatry. This also applied to Karl Peter Kisker (1926–1997), who became the first chair in psychiatry of the newly founded Hanover Medical School in 1966. There, he established a training course in social psychiatry. The training course was aimed not only at nurses, but at all professions dealing with psychiatry. This special, comprehensive orientation was based on Kisker's demand to create on the long run a new type of social psychiatric occupation, which he called "socio-therapist" or "sociagouge". The article deals with the question how Karl Peter Kisker as one of the main figures of early psychiatric reforms viewed the shortcomings of psychiatric nursing, how he formulated his demands for the future role of psychiatric nurses, and how he intended to put that role into practise.

Nurses as a subject of psychiatric reforms in Western Germany

In 1967, the teacher Frank Fischer was working for eight month in five psychiatric state hospitals in the Federal Republic of Germany as an assistant nurse. His aim was, in his own words, to "uncover" the "true character" of the asylum. He assumed that professional psychiatrists were lacking "the precise knowledge" of what was happening in the wards during their absence. The results of his covert participant observation were published in 1969 in the book "Asylums – The ill accuse" (*Irrenhäuser – Kranke klagen an*) which became very popular in Western Germany.[1]

At a time when the translation of important foreign books criticising psychiatry into German language boomed, such as Michel Foucault's *Madness and Society* (*Wahnsinn und Gesellschaft*, 1961/1969), Franco Basaglia's *L'istituzione negata* (*Die negierte Institution*, 1968/1971)[2], Ronald D. Laing's *The Divided Self* (*Das geteilte Selbst*, 1960/1972), Erving Goffman's *Asylums* (*Asyle*, 1961/1973) and also Ken Kesey's famous prose work *One flew over the cuckoo's nest* (*Einer flog über das Kuckucksnest*, 1962/1972), "madness" was becoming political topic and a public theme. The public image of a custodial psychiatry neglecting and humiliating its patients was at the same time closely connected to a certain

---

1   Fischer (1972).
2   Basaglia's work is still not translated into English. As the historian John Foot notes, "there are no convincing explanations of this non-translation, although there are various accounts available." See Foot (2015), p. 60.

image of the psychiatric nurse. Focussing the "non-medical surrounding" of institutional psychiatry, Fischer's book, too, described the nurses appearing as the "unrelenting administrators", "mechanical prison wardens" and "true rulers" of the clinic, with a "rattling bunch of keys to signal permanently who is the master of the house"[3].

At the same time, the early psychiatric reformers of the Department of Psychiatry at Heidelberg University – Walter v. Baeyer (1904–1987), Karl Peter Kisker, and Heinz Häfner (*1926)[4] – were highlighted by Fischer as positive examples of psychiatrists, who "tirelessly" pointed out the "totally inadequate psychiatric care" to their professional colleagues and the public[5]. For the cases of Heidelberg and Mannheim, their aims of reform also included initiatives to qualify nurses for a social psychiatry defined by psychiatrists who had to face that they were not the "masters of the clinic".

The Masters of the Clinic was the title of the covert participant observation by Rolf Dieter Hemprich and Karl Peter Kisker in the psychiatric clinic at Heidelberg University which was published just a few months before Fischer's book in October 1968.[6] Following similar studies like the US-American work *The mental hospital* by Alfred H. Stanton and Morris S. Schwartz from the 1954[7], it exemplified the colliding views on psychiatric work between "traditional" nursing and "progressive" psychiatric therapy. Stanton and Schwartz coined the term of "the other 23 hours", which Hemprich and Kisker and also Frank Fischer picked up in their studies. This term questioned the therapeutic control of the psychiatrists in their clinic beyond their visits in the wards. It seemed as if, with an upcoming new generation of social psychiatrists in Germany, the nurses' qualification for a re-defined psychiatric care was regarded as a considerable obstacle for the transformation of this care. These young psychiatrists of the 1960ies had not only to argue with their psychiatric teachers and supervisors, but also with a nursing staff used to support a custodial, patriarchal and secluded system of psychiatric care.

This article will describe how the medical professional vision and practise of a specific additional social psychiatric training developed in the lift-off-phase of psychiatric reforms in Federal Germany from the mid-1960s to the mid-1970s. For this it will focus on the example of the social psychiatric training in Hanover. First, it will start with Karl Peter Kisker's definition of the demands of professional training in social psychiatry, than it will describe the basic conditions of its realisation at the psychiatric department at the Hanover Medical School. Then the Hanover Medical School as "island of reform" will be regarded in its wider context of the status of nursing in psychiatry in Federal Germany in the 1970s.

---

3   Fischer (1972), p. 18, 40, 59.
4   See Maike Rotzoll in this book.
5   Fischer (1972), p. 141. For the role of Frank Fischer's book for the discussion of psychiatric reforms in the Federal Republic of Germany see Brink (2010), pp. 444–450.
6   Hemprich/Kisker (1968).
7   Stanton/Schwartz (1954).

A Psychiatric Department as a "training camp": Karl Peter Kisker in Hanover

The Hanover Medical School was newly founded in 1966 as a reform-orientated academy for medicine. Therefore it was not surprising that the Medical school chose Karl Peter Kisker as its first chair in psychiatry. As a representative of a phenomenological and anthropologic approach to mental illness, Kisker tried to bring out the meaningfulness and the situational coping with life characterising diseases like schizophrenia. The dialogue with the schizophrenic patient had to be resumed to train the co-existence with mentally deviant people through serene and persistent reflexion.[8] This approach to psychiatric illnesses led Karl Peter Kisker to a practical vision of the developing new occupation of "socio-therapists". As a consequence, Kisker established a professional training course in social psychiatry at the Medical School Hanover. This training was meant to be the first step to a new kind of therapeutical "mediators" he had already imagined in the study "Masters of the Clinic". In this article, Kisker and Hemprich described these future "mediators" as "true advisors" for the "everyday concerns" of the patients, with the intelligence and "mature personality" to work in every clinic and out-patient psychiatric service.[9]

The period of the professional training course at the Hanover Medical School was two years, encompassing one thousand hours of lessons. It included, amongst other things, participation in self-awareness groups, medical group therapies and policlinic family work, preparation and carrying out of cultural activities, advice of the newly-established patients committees, chairing of patients clubs and round of talks. The final exams consisted of one written assignment, two written tests, and two oral tests.[10] Proposals of topics for written tests in 1970 were, for example: "The mentally disabled in the view of society", "Therapeutic elements of situation games", "Considerations on the rehabilitation of the schizophrenic", "Tasks and problems of hospital care" and "Social and medical aspects of mental disability".[11] This first curriculum of the social psychiatric training in 1967 proves in detail the get-up-and-go attitude of early reformers in German psychiatry, placing a special emphasis on the role of society and family for mental diseases and searching an individual approach to the patient.

As Kisker stated in an exposé called "Present state and possibilities of development of education in social psychiatry" in 1970, the aim of "such an demanding education [...] will unquestionably be a new type of profession"

---

8   Schwarz (2015); Kisker (1976), on p. IV.
9   Hemprich/Kisker (1968), p. 441. At the same time, the authors denied that the nurses involved in their study met the "psychological minimum requirements" to become a "mediator".
10   Lehranstalt für Sozialpsychiatrische Zusatzausbildung an der MHH (1973), p. 77.
11   Anonymous (1973), p. 63.

besides the nurse or the social education worker[12], persons who will independently work on a regular basis in the social psychiatric team or in the management of social psychiatric services. In Kisker's application for the official recognition of the training course by the federal state of Lower Saxony, he also argued that the social shift in psychiatry would add prominence to "activating psycho- and socio-therapeutic ways of care". To meet "international standards" in education, the training programme at the Medical School would serve the need for socio-therapeutic personnel being capable of acting "independently and responsibly".[13]

These statements indicate that the start of the professional training in social psychiatry at Hanover Medical School was as experimental and provisional as the psychiatric department itself. Kisker himself later called the clinic of this department a "training camp".[14] In 1967, the psychiatric clinic opened on the grounds of the mental hospital in Wunstorf 30 kilometres from Hanover City centre because the buildings for the department of psychiatry at the medical school were still under construction. Projected as a "model institution to test socio-therapeutic measures", the purpose of the clinic containing three wards for 36 patients was the "re-integration of mentally ill that had been hospitalised for months and years"[15]. Therefore, the first patients of this clinic were "long-term patients" of the Wunstorf mental hospital.

These "long-term patients" were hand-picked according to their ability to take part in "socio-therapeutic" methods such as the "therapeutic community", a participative concept adapted from Maxwell Jones including milieu therapy, group psychotherapy and practical activities[16]. In that way, the new clinic distinguished itself from the everyday work at Wunstorf mental hospital which was characterized by the pitiful conditions of psychiatry in Western Germany at that time. Recognised as a "noble psychiatric ghetto"[17], the psychiatric branch of the Hanover Medical School at Wunstorf mainly took care of well-educated and young patients. With self-confidence as the spearheads of progressive social psychiatry the therapists of the clinic looked disdainfully at the outmoded mental hospital surrounding them. One quite typical result of those early dynamics of modernising psychiatry was the neglect of patients who were not able to take part in new methods such as the "therapeutic community". Therefore, in this early period the "drive" of the new clinic "missed out those patients that needed it the most".[18]

After a few years in this transitional phase, the "therapeutic community" at Wunstorf seemed to come to a dead end. The senior physician Helmut Krueger described his impressions of the "community" in 1970 in retrospec-

12 Kisker: Derzeitiger Stand (1973), p. 12.
13 Kisker: Antrag (1973), p. 51.
14 Kisker/Wulff (1985), p. 373.
15 Hofer (1967), p. 361.
16 For the role and development of this therapeutic instrument in psychiatry after World War II see for example Fussinger (2011).
17 Wittrock (2005), p. 132.
18 Finzen (1985), p. 55.

tive as a "therapeutic island" in danger of establishing an abnormal, ideological "subculture" in the psychiatric system. The patients appeared to him as a "crowd of noisy, scruffy [...] noble deadbeats lacking distance and respect for the therapist". At the same time, the therapists themselves seemed to doubt "the possibility of integrating psychiatric patients in this morbid capitalist society. Numerous discussions revealed the will to overcome the psychiatric institution itself, which could only be achieved by overcoming the societal conditions."[19]

It was therefore a crucial break when in 1972 the clinic moved from the grounds of the Wunstorf Mental Hospital to the now completed, new campus of Hanover Medical School. This relocation of the clinic also marked a shift from the experimental and exclusive phase of social psychiatry to a more open and pragmatic approach to psychiatric care. Since 1970 psychiatrists of the Hanover Medical School had been working on a concept of "community care", based on regional sectors inspired by the complex psychiatric community care systems existing in England at the London Maudsley Hospital.[20] In cooperation with the other psychiatric hospitals in the region, the psychiatric clinic of the Hanover Medical School in 1972 became the first university psychiatric department in Germany to assume the obligation for the admission of people in its sector. The system contained social psychiatric services and outreach clinics, day clinics, night clinics (1972), homes for people with disabilities (1970) and sheltered workshops (1973). By establishing this system, the Hanover Medical School was thus ahead of its time in Germany, and the so-called "Modell Hannover" became the first area-wide concept for psychiatric care in a large German city.

Nurse education and psychiatric reforms in the early 1970s

This development also had an impact on the training programme. The psychiatrist and manager of the training programme in Hanover in the early years Gregor Bosch described this change in the special issue "education" of the journal *Social Psychiatric informations* (*Sozialpsychiatrische Informationen*) in 1972, the programmes took a shift from a psychoanalytic "training in self-experience and perception of others [*Fremderfahrung*]" towards a more modest and practically based demand.[21]

Nevertheless, the path towards a more modest practise also had its conflicts. One focus of the criticism of social psychiatrists was the government-approved education of nurses revised in 1972, which included still no mandatory unit in psychiatric practice. The "dreadful state of education in psychiatry",

---

19 Krüger (1987), p. 17. A mainly positive patient's perspective of the therapeutic work at the Hanover Medical School Psychiatric Department at the Wunstorf Hospital gives Lindner (1994), pp. 28–29.
20 Werner-Kneißl (2009), p. 3.
21 Bosch (1973), p. 4.

like Gregor Bosch had phrased it, resulted especially from the lack of "functioning and sufficient social psychiatric model fields" at the federal state psychiatric hospitals.[22]

The nurse's training as it was therefore appeared to the educational reformers as "narrow education".[23] But the Hanover training course was also criticised for educating nurses, social workers, occupational therapists, physiotherapists and related professions together. Like Wiltrud Häfner-Ranabaur as the head of the training programme at the Psychiatric department of the Heidelberg University pointed out in 1970, this would lead to a "confusion of roles in the therapeutic milieu" and to rivalries between "just seemingly equal therapeutic professions".[24] Peter Bastiaan, head of the training programme in Hanover from 1975 to 2007, described in retrospective that these rivalries mainly existed between work therapists or ergotherapists and nurses. In his view, it affected mainly the group work with patients during the training. The occupational therapists thought that they were better prepared for this than nurses because the latter had no practise in group work through their former apprenticeship.[25]

In this context it is worthy of consideration, that these social psychiatric training courses required as a precondition a nurse training approved by the state, which was by no means usual in psychiatry in the federal republic of Germany. The final report of the so-called *Psychiatrie-Enquete* statet in 1975, that just 42 percent of the nurses working in in-patient psychiatry had passed such an exam and just six percent had completed a training course for social psychiatry. In comparison, more than fifty percent of all people working as nurses in psychiatry were employed as nursing helpers (17,4%), in education (16,8%) or without any education in nursing (17%).[26] In state hospitals there were 15 times more nurses working than in university clinics. But twice as many nurses working in university clinics than nurses in state hospitals took social psychiatric training courses.[27]

With regard to these numbers it seems not surprising that Fritz Reimer, head of the state hospital Weinsberg close to Heidelberg, stated in 1974 that nurses are "poisoned" "by the "principle of custodian care" in the state hospitals, overburdened by jobs outside of their profession such as cleaning the wards, serving the meals, counting clothes and so on. Reimer wrote in 1974, that cleaners and chronically ill patients could do such jobs "just as well" as nurses.[28] This refers to the close connection between working conditions, clinic structure and profession groups, which could lead to very practical obstacles of reform in every day nursing of a state hospital. Furthermore, such

---

22   Bosch (1973), p. 4.
23   Häfner-Ranabaur (1973), p. 102.
24   Häfner-Ranabaur (1973), p. 103.
25   Phone Interview with Peter Bastiaan, 24.9.2015.
26   Deutscher Bundestag (1975), p. 12.
27   Deutscher Bundestag (1975), pp. 129–131.
28   Reimer (1971), p. 325.

statements depict the change in the psychiatrist's view as to what the profession of psychiatric nursing should be. Following Fritz Reimer, nurses "unable to adjust" to the social psychiatry must be transferred. But their "once learned and trained abilities" are still useful and would fit "quite good" in geriatric wards.[29]

This suggestion exemplifies not only the trenches between views of "traditional" and "progressive" nursing, but also the difference between the reform ideals at university clinics and the pragmatism at state hospitals in Federal Germany. This was mentioned as a problem in the professional training in Hanover. The head of the programme Peter Bastiaan wrote in 1979, that nurses coming from other hospitals had difficulties in putting into practise what they learn at the Medical School. Self-experience should lead them to a view of the patient as a "human with problems in his life, but not as the 'completely other' and 'madmen'".[30] Obstacles of putting this into practise depended on the lack of support of their higher authorities, psychiatrists and colleagues at the psychiatric hospitals. This even included exemption from duty for nurses of the state hospitals participating in the programme[31] or the disapproval of implementing cultural activities in long-term-patient wards.[32] Therefore, improvements by nurses who had completed the training programme varied widely: from making "talking to the patients more popular" in the clinic to organising outpatient care.[33] In a survey 17 out of 146 graduates of the Hanover training programme named as biggest source of disappointment the failure of achieving changes. So in 1983 Peter Bastiaan had to ask, "if the social psychiatric training programme evokes too big hopes regarding the psychiatric work and reflects the implementation too little"[34].

Conclusion

To conclude, these last remarks highlight the question of nurses taking an active part in reforming psychiatric institutions – a topic which is rarely investigated in the history of german psychiatry.[35] In the 1960s, the role of the nurses in psychiatric hospitals became – with regard to the history of psychiatric nursing, we can say once again – a problem discussed by medical professionals. At the same time, the reports about the inhumane conditions in psychiatric state hospitals in Federal Germany increased. Covert participant observation from the nurse's perspective played a significant role both in popular and

---

29   Reimer (1971), p. 325.
30   Bastiaan/Vesenbeckh (1979), p. 215.
31   Bastiaan/Vesenbeckh (1979), p. 209.
32   Phone Interview with Peter Bastiaan, 24.9.2015.
33   Bastiaan (1983), 67.
34   Bastiaan (1983), 69.
35   An exception is for example the role of the personnel in scandalising the conditions in the Alsterdorf Institution in Hamburg, Engelbracht/Hauser (2013), pp. 281–298.

scientific criticism of the asylums. The German historian Cornelia Brink pointed out that the history of the psychiatric reforms in Germany "basically remained the business of the former medical protagonists of the movement"[36]. How nurses took part in setting reforms in motion is still an extensively open question which needs further research.

One option was to take part in training programmes such as the one established by Karl Kisker at Hanover Medical School. The development of these trainings in social psychiatry was based on the psychiatrist's experience of nurses not being able or not willing to take part in new models such as "therapeutic communities", "patient committees", cultural activities for the patients and so on. But: the motivation of nurses to attend these additional training programmes for social psychiatry gives a hint of a different attitude of them towards caring coming from the "basis". Of course another reason might have been, for example, the option to getting better wages after having successfully completed the course in Hanover.[37]

Like the training course in Heidelberg, the Hanover programme also implied in a way a new nursing "elite", mainly working in leading positions in a system of social psychiatric care. In the case of Hanover, this is for example indicated by the fact that no more than sixteen to twenty nurses were admitted to each training programme, and that they were mainly coming from the Medical School itself. The "sociagogue" as profession projected by Kisker was in the end not realised – also because of the specialties of the German Psychiatric Reform, which did not lead to a fundamental questioning of the once established psychiatric system, with the hospital remaining in its centre. Therefore, the problem as well as the media image of the psychiatric nurse as guard "with a rattling bunch of keys" also remained.

Bibliography

Printed sources

Anonymous: Zusatzausbildung Hannover: Themen der Klausurarbeiten. In: Sozialpsychiatrische Informationen, Sonderheft "Ausbildungs-Info", April 1973, pp. 63–66.
Bastiaan, Peter: Die Sozialpsychiatrische Zusatzausbildung an der Medizinischen Hochschule Hannover. In: Sozialpsychiatrische Informationen 2 (1983), pp. 56–76.
Bastiaan, Peter; Vesenbeckh, W.: Die sozialpsychiatrische Zusatzausbildung an der Medizinischen Hochschule Hannover (SPZA). In: Psychiatrische Praxis 4 (1979), pp. 207–220.
Bosch, Gregor: Zur Einführung. In: Sozialpsychiatrische Informationen, Sonderheft "Ausbildungs-Info", April 1973, pp. 2–8.

---

36 Brink (2010), p. 370.
37 Graduates of the social psychiatric training programme of the Hanover Medical School were getting a better pay scale than other nurses in Lower Saxony, even when those completed courses for special psychiatric nursing [psychiatrische Fachkrankenpflege]. Bastiaan (1983), p. 56.

Deutscher Bundestag: Bericht über die Lage der Psychiatrie in der Bundesrepublik Deutsch-
    land. Zur psychiatrischen und psychotherapeutisch/psychosomatischen Versorgung der
    Bevölkerung. Bundestagsdrucksache 7/4200. Bonn 1975.
Häfner-Ranabaur, Wiltrud: Diskussionsbemerkung. In: Sozialpsychiatrische Informationen,
    Sonderheft "Ausbildungs-Info", April 1973, pp. 102–105.
Hemprich, Rolf D.; Kisker, Karl P.: Die "Herren der Klinik" und die Patienten. Erfahrungen
    aus der teilnehmend-verdeckten Beobachtung einer psychiatrischen Station. In: Der Ner-
    venarzt 10 (1968), pp. 433–441.
Hofer, Georg: Aufbau und Gestalt der psychiatrischen Klinik. In: Niedersächsisches Ärzte-
    blatt 11 (1967), pp. 360–362.
Kisker, Karl P.: Antrag auf staatliche Anerkennung einer sozialpsychiatrischen Fachausbil-
    dung für Krankenschwestern, Krankenpfleger, Sozialarbeiter, Beschäftigungstherapeutin-
    nen, Pädagogen, usw. an den Herrn Kultusminister des Landes Niedersachsen, vom
    13.2.1968. In: Sozialpsychiatrische Informationen, Sonderheft "Ausbildungs-Info", April
    1973, pp. 51–55.
Kisker, Karl P.: Derzeitiger Stand und Entwicklungsmöglichkeiten für Sozialpsychiatrische
    Ausbildungen. In: Sozialpsychiatrische Informationen, Sonderheft "Ausbildungs-Info",
    April 1973, pp. 11–14.
Kisker, Karl P.: Mit den Augen eines Psychiaters. Stuttgart 1976.
Lehranstalt für Sozialpsychiatrische Zusatzausbildung an der MHH: Merkblatt zur Sozialpsy-
    chiatrischen Zusatzausbildung 1972. In: Sozialpsychiatrische Informationen, Sonderheft
    "Ausbildungs-Info", April 1973, pp. 74–77.
Reimer, Fritz: Personalprobleme im psychiatrischen Krankenhaus. In: Deutsche Kranken-
    pflegezeitschrift 24 (1971), pp. 324–326.

Secondary research literature

Brink, Cornelia: Grenzen der Anstalt. Psychiatrie und Gesellschaft in Deutschland 1860–
    1980. Göttingen 2010.
Engelbracht, Gerda; Hauser, Andrea: Mitten in Hamburg. Die Alsterdorfer Anstalten 1945–
    1979. Stuttgart 2013.
Finzen, Asmus: Das Ende der Anstalt. Vom mühsamen Alltag der Reformpsychiatrie. Bonn
    1985.
Fischer, Frank: Irrenhäuser. Kranke klagen an. München; Wien; Basel 1972.
Foot, John: The Man Who Closed the Asylums. Franco Basaglia and the Revolution in Men-
    tal Health Care. London; New York 2015.
Fussinger, Catherine: "Therapeutic Community", Psychiatry's Reformers and Antipsychia-
    trists: Reconsidering Changes in the Field of Psychiatry after World War II. In: History of
    Psychiatry 22 (2011), pp. 146–163.
Kisker, Karl Peter; Wulff, Erich: Psychiatrie. In: Rektor der Medizinischen Hochschule Han-
    nover (ed.): Medizinische Hochschule Hannover 1965–1985. Hannover 1985, pp. 372–
    380.
Krüger, Heinrich: Reifungskrisen einer Klinik: Anti-institutionelles Wollen und Therapeuti-
    sche Gemeinschaft. In: Haselbeck, Heinz et al. (ed): Psychiatrie in Hannover. Struktur-
    wandel und therapeutische Praxis in einem gemeindenahen Versorgungssystem. Stuttgart
    1987, pp. 16–23.
Lindner, Heidi: Viele Tode stirbt der Mensch. Autobiographie mit Träumen und Erlebnissen
    einer psychisch kranken Frau. Gütersloh 1994.
Schwarz, Julian: Kisker, Karl Peter. In: Biographisches Archiv der Psychiatrie. URL: www.
    biapsy.de/index.php/de/9-biographien-a-z/103-kisker-karl-peter (22.08.2016).

Stanton, Alfred H.; Schwartz, Morris S.: The Mental Hospital. A Study of Institutional Partici-
    pation in Psychiatric Illness and Treatment. New York 1954.
Werner-Kneißl, Johann: Lebensräume – Wie alles begann. Interview with Manfred Bauer. In:
    Lebensräume, 1.1.2009, pp. 1–9.
Wittrock, Heinrich: Niedersächsisches Landeskrankenhaus Wunstorf. Von der Korrektions-
    anstalt zum modernen Fachkrankenhaus (1880–2005). Wunstorf 2005.

List of Authors

Christof Beyer, Dr.
Institut für Geschichte, Ethik und Philosophie der Medizin
Medizinische Hochschule Hannover
Carl-Neuberg-Str. 1
30625 Hannover
Beyer.Christof@mh-hannover.de

Geertje Boschma, PhD, RN, Professor
School of Nursing
University of British Columbia
T201–2211 Wesbrook Mall, Vancouver BC V6T 2B5
geertje.boschma@nursing.ubc.ca

Sabine Braunschweig, Dr.
Büro für Sozialgeschichte
Dornacherstrasse 192
CH-4053 Basel, Switzerland
braunschweig@sozialgeschichte-bs.ch

Mary B. Connell, MScN
School of Nursing
Faculty of Health Sciences
University of Ottawa
451 Smyth Raod
Ottawa ON K1H 8M5
Mconn031@uottawa.ca

Åshild Fause, RN, Phd, Associate Professor
Department of Health and Care Sciences
The Faculty of Health Sciences
UIT Norwegian Arctic University
9037 Tromsø, Norway
Ashild.fause@uit.no

Thomas Foth, RN, MScN, MA(Ed), PhD
Université d'Ottawa / University of Ottawa
Faculté des sciences de la santé / Faculty of Health sciences
Écoles des sciences infirmières / School of Nursing
451 Smyth Road
Ottawa, Ontario
Canada
K1H 8M5
thomas.foth@uottawa.ca

Jens Gründler, Dr.
Fachbereich Geschichtswissenschaft der Universität Tübingen
Seminar für Neuere Geschichte
Wilhelmstraße 36
72074 Tübingen
jensgruendler@mac.com

Sylvelyn Hähner-Rombach, Dr.
Institut für Geschichte der Medizin der Robert Bosch Foundation
Straussweg 17
D-70184 Stuttgart
Sylvelyn.haehner@igm-bosch.de

Sandra Harrisson, inf. PhD (c.)
Professeure
Université du Québec à Trois-Rivières
Département des Sciences Infirmières
3351, boul. des Forges
C. P. 500
Trois-Rivières (Québec) G 9A 5 H7
sandra.harrisson@uqtr.ca

Jette Lange, PhD
School of Nursing
Faculty of Health Sciences
University of Ottawa
451 Smyth Raod
Ottawa ON K1H 8M5
Jlang102@uottawa.ca

Cheryl S. McWatters, PhD, Associate Prof.
Telfer School of Business
University of Ottawa
55 Laurier Ave E
Ottawa ON K1N 6N5
mcwatters@telfer.uottawa.ca

Karen Nolte, PD Dr.
Institut für Geschichte der Medizin
Universität Würzburg
Oberer Neubergweg 10 a
97074 Würzburg
karen.nolte@uni-wuerzburg.de

Maike Rotzoll, PD Dr.
Institut für Geschichte und Ethik der Medizin
Martin-Luther-Universität Halle-Wittenberg
Magdeburger Str. 8
06112 Halle/Saale
maike.rotzoll@medizin.uni-halle.de

Institut für Geschichte und Etik der Medizin
Ruprecht-Karls-Universität Heidelberg
Im Neuenheimer Feld 327
69120 Heidelberg
maike.rotzoll@histmed.uni-heidelberg.de

MEDIZIN, GESELLSCHAFT UND GESCHICHTE — BEIHEFTE

Herausgegeben von Robert Jütte.

Franz Steiner Verlag   ISSN 0941–5033